Mini Pig Natural Diet Guide
The AMPA's Ultimate Cookbook of Healthy Meals & Treats

Stephanie Matlock & Kimberly Chronister

CONTENTS

INTRODUCTION

The Mini Pig Natural Diet Guide is designed as a reference only. Feeding amounts and portion sizes vary with the needs of the individual pig. The following recipes may be incorporated into any diet. Portion each recipe into the number of servings appropriate for your pig. Treat your mini pig with special home cooked meals to replace an occasional pelleted meal or transform the health of your mini pig with a completely natural diet. A complete diet includes a variety of grains, seeds, nuts, vegetables, and occasional fruit. Vitamins and supplements may be added to ensure nutritional needs are met. Always consult your veterinarian if you have any questions or concerns about your mini pig's health or nutritional needs.

CHAPTER 1

Beginner's Guide to Healthy Mini Pig Diet

Feeding mini pigs a healthy, nutritious diet can be simple, fun, and interesting. Most new pig parents choose to feed commercial mini pig pellets to their pigs while they learn about more natural choices. These specially formulated foods have most of the nutrients a pig needs, but also usually have a few unnecessary cheap filler foods. A pelleted diet supplemented with healthy foods and grazing is a top choice for many families. Healthy recipes from this book can be added or supplemented to these diets.

Commonly available brands of food are Mazuri Mini Pig, Manna Pro Mini Pig, Purina Nature's Match Pig & Sow, Nutrena Country Feeds Mini Pig, and Sharp's Mini Pig Food (available online only). Each brand has slightly different ingredients, nutritional offerings, and meal sizes. Mini pig pellets may be found at local farm stores. Tractor Supply, Orscheln, Atwoods, and Rural King usually carry mini pig pellets or can special order them.

The general recommendation for daily pellet requirements by Dr. Cathy Corrigan is approximately ½ cup pellets per 25 lbs body weight or 1-2% of body weight, split up into an appropriate number of meals each day. The genetics, environment, and dietary needs of each pig varies between individuals, making this a starting point only. Adjust daily food intake as you gauge your pig's own needs. They may need more or less than the standard amount.

In addition to the pelleted portion of the diet, mini pigs benefit from heaping servings of dark leafy greens, healthy vegetables, occasional snacks or training treats, as well as grazing and foraging in the yard. All these additions in the diet add to the caloric load and should be offered in moderation for a healthy, balanced diet. Grazing is particularly nutrient dense. If offered plenty of grazing time or extra snacks, then the pelleted portion of the diet may need to be adjusted to compensate for the extra calories consumed in other parts of the diet.

When putting together a diet plan for your mini pig, keep in mind their nutritional needs.

Pigs are unique animals in the way they can grow and gain weight rapidly with relatively small amounts of food. They require a low protein diet with high fiber. Pellets and grains should be limited with larger portions of dark leafy greens and healthy vegetables. Staple choices to add moisture and dietary bulk to meals are spinach, romaine, beet greens, mustard greens, kale, chard, bok choy, arugula, dandelion greens, summer squashes, winter squashes, cherry tomatoes, parsnips, broccoli, sweet potatoes, eggplant, beets, rutabagas, turnips, celery, and peas. Alternatively, choose healthy salad recipes in this book, topping with a serving of pellets for a nutritionally completely and satisfying meal.

To help pigs get more enjoyment and more fulfilling meals, offer enrichment activities. These activities help nurture the pig's body and mind by providing physical exercise and mental stimulation while slowing down their meal. Treat dispensing toys and scattering meals in the yard gives the pigs a chance to use their natural foraging instincts and powerful rooting snout to find their food.

Shaping a dietary plan to meet a mini pig's nutritional needs is a balancing act of give and take. If given the chance, they will quickly eat themselves into painful & debilitating obesity. As caretakers of these amazing animals, it is our responsibility to control and manage the portions to keep them at a healthy weight for a long, active, healthy life.

What makes a good pet pig diet?

Cathy (Zolicani) Corrigan, DVM

06/13/2017

There are several factors that must be considered before selecting a diet for your small breed of pig. Our goal is to provide our pet pigs with superior nutrition for a long and disease-free life. We must consider the basic nutritional requirements of the pig, ease of production and storage, origin of ingredients, bioavailabiity, the energy needs of the pig, palatability, ease of feeding, price, and access to the product.

1. Basic nutritional requirements

The basic nutritional needs of our small breeds of pigs (for adults) include:

Protein % 13-16

Fat % 3.5

Fiber % 14

Calcium % 0.95

phosphorus % 0.80

Selenium ppm 0.48

Zn ppm 140

Vitamin A (IU/kg) 6000

Vitamin E (IU/kg) 180

Vitamin D (IU/kg) 1120

2. Ease of production and storage

A homemade diet with completely fresh ingredients would be ideal for all of us – but homemade diets that are balanced for a pig are time consuming, difficult to make, and expensive.

A pre-packaged diet, covering the basic nutritional needs, but supplemented with a variety of fresh foods and graze is a reasonable compromise. There are many pelleted diets available for pigs. Most of them cover the basic requirements, but many are produced for production pigs and may not meet our standards for a pet pig's diet.

3. Origin of ingredients

This is when it begins to get complicated.

The larger food companies often buy ingredients on the commodity market…corn may be substituted for barley because corn is cheaper at that time. OR corn from China or Chile may be cheaper than locally grown corn. Care may not be taken to make sure the product is not contaminated with toxins (like the melamine contamination in dog foods causing kidney failure) or is not a GMO product.

The soil used to grow the ingredients may also be depleted of certain nutrients – either due to over use or because of the geography. The soil in the pacific northwest of the United States has almost no selenium or magnesium, so grains or hays grown in this area do not provide adequate levels of these nutrients when eaten.

Shelf life is a factor also – the longer the product stays on the shelf, the more nutrients leak out of the food due to oxidation. Contamination from moisture, mold, rodents, and bugs is also more likely.

4. Bioavailability

This involves the ability of the pig to digest and absorb nutrients from the food. Some pigs do not have the digestive enzymes and intestinal flora to absorb nutrients. Foods that contain preservatives or have fewer nutrients are harder for these pigs to digest.

Fresher ingredients are usually, but not always, easier for a pig to digest. The more nutrient-dense a product is, the more likely that the pig will be able to utilize it. Production and preservation tend to dilute nutrients or render them unusable.

Another factor to bioavailability is the ratio of nutrients and their use in the body. The Calcium/Phosphorus ration of foods is critical, especially to young growing pigs, or to the elderly pigs, who may be developing bone disease. The dietary requirements of Calcium:Phosphorus should be 1.2 (Ca):1(phosphorus). Appropriate levels of Vitamin A and D must also be available to utilize these minerals properly. In addition, other foods can alter the metabolism. In a condition call bran sickness, too much wheat bran is fed. The wheat bran has a very large amount of phosphorus in it. The "overdose" of phosphorus causes the calcium to leach out of the bone, and the bones spontaneously fracture. This is called nutritional hyperparathyroidism or Nutritional Osteodystrophy.

5. Energy needs of the pig

Young, growing pigs need more food. Creep feeding (having food spread out in the pig enclosure for piglets to root and find – small amounts constantly available through the day) any diet is necessary for growing piglets.

Active pigs need more food than inactive pigs.

Obese pigs need less food (and more activity). These pigs still need a BALANCED diet, just less of the food.

6. Palatability

If a pig will not eat the food, or if they eat only parts of it, but not the total diet, then they are not getting a balanced diet.

7. Ease of feeding

A dry packaged food is easy to feed, easy to store, easy to find and buy.

8. Price

Large batch commercial foods are usually quite reasonably priced.

Small batch, local foods are more expensive, but often are more nutritious. They may be harder to find.

9. Access to the product.

Not much of an issue due to the internet. Except for handmade diets, which can be difficult.

CHAPTER 2

7 DAY MEAL PLAN

Feeding amounts vary with the needs of the individual pig. Feed amounts according to body condition. Vegetables and grains make up the bulk of the mini pig's diet with nuts, seeds, and trail mix accounting for a small portion. Listed weekly meal plans include 3 meals per day for convenience. You may condense this plan into two meals per day by adjusting amounts of breakfast and dinner.

Basic Weekly Menu Plan

Sunday

Breakfast - AMPA Natural Diet Grains Mixture (cooked), leafy greens, choice of drink (optional)

Lunch – Choice of salad sprinkled with AMPA Mini Pig Seed Mix, Mini Pig Trail Mix for enrichment activity

Dinner - AMPA Natural Diet Grains Mixture (cooked), choice of side vegetables

Monday

Breakfast - AMPA Natural Diet Grains Mixture (cooked), 1 egg scrambled with spinach

Lunch – Choice of salad, choice of smoothie (optional), AMPA Mini Pig Seed Mix for enrichment activity

Dinner – AMPA Natural Diet Grains Mixture (cooked), side salad

Tuesday

Breakfast – Cooked oatmeal, black oil sunflower seeds, diced pumpkin or squash

Lunch - Choice of salad sprinkled with AMPA Mini Pig Seed Mix, choice of drink (optional), AMPA Natural Diet Dry Mixture for enrichment activity

Dinner - AMPA Natural Diet Grains Mixture (cooked), side salad, choice of soup (optional)

Wednesday

Breakfast- AMPA Natural Diet Grains Mixture (cooked), side salad with cranberries, infused water

Lunch - Choice of salad sprinkled with AMPA Mini Pig Seed Mix, AMPA Mini Pig Trail Mix for enrichment activity

Dinner - AMPA Natural Diet Grains Mixture (cooked), mixed vegetables,

Thursday

Breakfast - AMPA Natural Diet Grains Mixture (cooked), scrambled egg

Lunch - Choice of salad, AMPA Natural Diet Dry Mixture for enrichment activity

Dinner - AMPA Natural Diet Grains Mixture (cooked), side salad

Friday

Breakfast - AMPA Natural Diet Grains Mixture (cooked), diced vegetables

Lunch - Choice of salad sprinkled with AMPA Mini Pig Seed Mix, choice of drink (optional), AMPA Mini Pig Trail Mix for enrichment activity

Dinner - AMPA Natural Diet Grains Mixture (cooked), side salad, choice of dessert (optional)

Saturday

Breakfast - AMPA Natural Diet Grains Mixture (cooked), spinach, choice of drink (optional)

Lunch - Choice of salad, AMPA Natural Diet Dry Mixture for enrichment activity

Dinner - AMPA Natural Diet Grains Mixture (cooked), mixed vegetables, choice of soup (optional)

AMPA Natural Diet Grain Mixture (COOKED)– For Use In Multiple Recipes

Ingredients:

1 part brown rice

1 part lentils

1 part beans

1 part rolled oats

1 part barley

1 part wheat

Instructions:

Cook all foods per package directions. Once cooked and cooled, mix all ingredients together and store portion sizes in freezer for freshness. A large batch can be made and rationed out over time with the listed proportions. This has a higher protein content than the AMPA Natural Diet Dry Mixture (Enrichment) due to the lentils and beans. Serve appropriate portion as a meal or include in the following recipes.

AMPA Natural Diet Dry Mixture

Ingredients:

1 part wheat

1 part milo

1 part barley

1 part quinoa

1 part nuts & seeds: chia seeds, sesame seeds, almonds, pumpkin seeds, etc

1 part black oil sunflower seeds

2 parts rolled oats

Instructions:

Serve appropriate portion as a meal, incorporate into the following recipes, or use in enrichment activities for a meal on the go!

AMPA Mini Pig Trail Mix

Ingredients:

1 cup raw whole almonds

1 cup raw pumpkin seeds

1 cup black oil sunflower seeds

1 cup mix nuts, unsalted (almonds, peanut, walnuts, brazil nuts, cashews, hazelnuts, macadamia nuts, pine nuts

1 cup banana chips

Instructions:

Store in airtight container and use as appropriate.

AMPA Mini Pig Seed Mix

Ingredients:

1 cup black oil sunflower seeds

1 cup raw pumpkin seeds

1 cup sesame seeds

1 cup chia seeds

1 cup quinoa

Instructions:

Store in airtight container and use as appropriate.

Gourmet Week 1

Sunday

Breakfast – Peas and Carrots Mini Egg Cups, Coconut Cucumber Cooler

Lunch – Classic Kale Salad, AMPA Mini Pig Trail Mix for enrichment activity

Dinner – Slow Cooker Wheat Berries, side of spinach

Monday

Breakfast – Quinoa Fruity Salad, Cranberry Pumpkin Smoothie

Lunch – Roasted Vegetables, AMPA Mini Pig Trail Mix for enrichment activity

Dinner – AMPA Natural Diet Grain Mixture (cooked), side salad or mixed vegetables

Tuesday

Breakfast – Pumpkin Coconut Oatmeal, Pineapple Mint Infused Water

Lunch – Green Bean Salad, AMPA Mini Pig Trail Mix for enrichment activity

Dinner – Chickpea Tabbouleh, leafy greens

Wednesday

Breakfast – Apple Barley Breakfast, Cranberry Kale Smoothie

Lunch – Ginger Lentils, Swiss Chard Salad, AMPA Mini Pig Trail Mix for enrichment activity

Dinner – Fiesta Burrito Bowl

Thursday

Breakfast – Quinoa Breakfast Bowl, ACV Health Boosting Splash

Lunch – Cucumber Beet Salad, AMPA Mini Pig Trail Mix for enrichment activity

Dinner - AMPA Natural Diet Grain Mixture (cooked), side salad or mixed vegetables

Friday

Breakfast – Strawberry Almond Oatmeal, Melon Basil Infused Water

Lunch – Broccoli Stuffed Sweet Potato, AMPA Mini Pig Trail Mix for enrichment activity

Dinner – Eggplant Barley Dinner, Strawberry Mousse

Saturday

Breakfast - Barley Breakfast Bowl, Coconut Pumpkin Smoothie

Lunch – Cranberry Broccoli Salad, AMPA Mini Pig Trail Mix for enrichment activity

Dinner – Spaghetti Squash Dinner Bowl

Gourmet Week 2

Sunday

Breakfast – Quinoa Chia Porridge, Apple Cranberry UTI Buster

Lunch – Green Beans with Cranberries, AMPA Mini Pig Trail Mix for enrichment activity

Dinner - AMPA Natural Diet Grain Mixture (cooked), side salad or mixed vegetables

Monday

Breakfast – Scrambled Cauliflower, Almond Spinach Smoothie

Lunch – Zucchini & Corn Succotash, AMPA Mini Pig Trail Mix for enrichment activity

Dinner - Summer Grilled Burrito Bowl

Tuesday

Breakfast – Mini Veggie Frittatas, Raspberry Ginger Basil Infused Water

Lunch – Orange Pecan Spinach Salad, AMPA Mini Pig Trail Mix for enrichment activity

Dinner – Texas Caviar

Wednesday

Breakfast – Peach and Black Bean Salsa, Cranberry Coconut Refresher

Lunch – Nutty Butternut Squash, AMPA Mini Pig Trail Mix for enrichment activity

Dinner - AMPA Natural Diet Grain Mixture (cooked), side salad or mixed vegetables

Thursday

Breakfast - Barley Breakfast Bowl, Pumpkin Smoothie

Lunch – Warm Brussel Sprouts Quinoa Salad, AMPA Mini Pig Trail Mix for enrichment activity

Dinner - Pumpkin Puree Dinner

Friday

Breakfast – Make Ahead Pumpkin Oats, Watermelon Rosemary Infused Water

Lunch – Power Green Salad, AMPA Mini Pig Trail Mix for enrichment activity

Dinner – Lettuce Wrap Bowls, Fresh Breath Parsley Mint Parfait Bites

Saturday

Breakfast – Pumpkin Quinoa Quiche, Berries & Beets Smoothie

Lunch – Honey Roasted Parsnips & Carrots, AMPA Mini Pig Trail Mix for enrichment activity

Dinner - AMPA Natural Diet Grain Mixture (cooked), side salad or mixed vegetables

Gourmet Week 3

Sunday

Breakfast – Quinoa Chia Porridge, Refreshing Detox Infused Water

Lunch – Stir Fry Ginger Mustard Greens, AMPA Mini Pig Trail Mix for enrichment activity

Dinner – Stuffed Acorn Squash

Monday

Breakfast – Banana Clove Pancakes, Cool Mint Smoothie

Lunch – Blueberry Dandelion Salad, AMPA Mini Pig Trail Mix for enrichment activity

Dinner – Sprouted Lentils Dish

Tuesday

Breakfast - Make Ahead Pumpkin Oats, Blackberry Sage Infused Water

Lunch – Roasted Cauliflower and spinach, AMPA Mini Pig Trail Mix for enrichment activity

Dinner - AMPA Natural Diet Grain Mixture (cooked), side salad or mixed vegetables

Wednesday

Breakfast – Strawberry Almond Oatmeal, Hydration Therapy Smoothie

Lunch – Power Green Salad, AMPA Mini Pig Trail Mix for enrichment activity

Dinner – Eggplant Chickpea Bake

Thursday

Breakfast – Red & Green Mini Pig Egg Cup, Coconut Cucumber Infused Water

Lunch - Summer Fun Lunch, AMPA Mini Pig Trail Mix for enrichment activity

Dinner – Pumpkin Black Bean Salad

Friday

Breakfast – Zucchini Breakfast Bowl, Powerhouse Pumpkin Smoothie

Lunch – Black Bean Salad, AMPA Mini Pig Trail Mix for enrichment activity

Dinner - AMPA Natural Diet Grain Mixture (cooked), side salad or mixed vegetables, Pumpkin Pie Bites

Saturday

Breakfast – Pumpkin Coconut Oatmeal, Cranberry Coconut Refresher

Lunch – Cranberry Infused Brussel Sprouts with chopped or canned pumpkin

Dinner – Artichoke Stuffed Eggplant

Gourmet Week 4

Sunday

Breakfast – Banana Clove Pancakes, Coconut Cucumber Cooler

Lunch – Apple Cranberry Walnut Salad

Dinner – Egg Fried Rice & More

Monday

Breakfast – Broccoli Carrots Mini Egg Cup, Triple Berry Infused Water

Lunch – Spinach Pumpkin Salad, AMPA Mini Pig Trail Mix for enrichment activity

Dinner - AMPA Natural Diet Grain Mixture (cooked), side salad or mixed vegetables

Tuesday

Breakfast – Zucchini Breakfast Bowl, Pumpkin Smoothie

Lunch – Honey Glazed Carrots and Brussels Sprouts, AMPA Mini Pig Trail Mix for enrichment activity

Dinner – Loaded Sweet Potatoes

Wednesday

Breakfast - Sunny Side Up Salad, Blue Kiwi Infused Water

Lunch – Zucchini Corn Black Bean Mixup, AMPA Mini Pig Trail Mix for enrichment activity

Dinner – Stuffed Bell Peppers

Thursday

Breakfast – Baked Oatmeal Mini Pig Cups, ACV Health Boosting Splash

Lunch – Zucchini and Corn Succotash

Dinner - AMPA Natural Diet Grain Mixture (cooked), side salad or mixed vegetables

Friday

Breakfast – Apple Barley Breakfast, Apple Cranberry UTI Buster

Lunch – Coconut Roasted Baby Carrots, AMPA Mini Pig Trail Mix for enrichment activity

Dinner – Mushroom Rice Gourmet, Apple Crisp

Saturday

Breakfast – Scrambled Cauliflower, Berry Oat Smoothie

Lunch – Honey Roasted Parsnips & Carrots

Dinner – Spinach Rice Balls

CHAPTER 3

HEALTHY & TOXIC FOODS LIST

Vegetables:

- ALL summer & winter squash
- Acorn Squash
- Amaranth
- Arrowroot
- Artichoke
- Arugula
- Asparagus
- Banana Squash
- Bamboo shoots
- Beets
- Belgian endive
- Bell Peppers
- Black Eyed Peas
- Black olives (fed sparingly due to sodium content)
- Black Radish
- Black Salsify
- Bok choy
- Broccoli
- Brussels sprouts
- Burdock Root
- Butter Lettuce
- Buttercup Squash
- Butternut Squash
- Cabbage & red cabbage
- Carrots
- Cauliflower
- Celery Root
- Celery
- Chayote Squash
- Cherry Tomatoes
- Chickweed
- Chives
- Collard greens
- Corn (sparingly, there's enough corn in their pellets already)
- Cucumbers
- Dandelion flower and leaves

- Eggplant
- Endive
- Fava Beans
- Fennel
- Galangal Root
- Green Beans
- Green leaf lettuce
- Green Soybeans (Edamame)
- Jicama
- Kale
- Kohlrabi
- Leeks
- Lettuce
- Lima Beans
- Manoa
- Lettuce
- Mushrooms
- Mustard Greens
- Okra
- Olives
- Parsnips
- Pea Pods
- Peanuts (unsalted)
- Peas Plantain
- Pumpkin
- Purple Asparagus
- Radicchio
- Radishes & leaves
- Red clover
- Red Leaf Lettuce
- Rhubarb stem/stalk (the leaves are poisonous and should not be fed)
- Romaine lettuce
- Rutabagas
- Shallots
- Snow Peas
- Sorrel
- Spinach
- Spring Baby Lettuce
- Sugar Snap Peas
- Sweet Dumpling Squash
- Sweet Potatoes
- Swiss chard
- Tomatoes (tomatoes are good but the plant and leaves are poisonous and should not be fed)
- Turnip greens
- Turnips
- Wasabi Root
- Watercress
- Winged Beans
- Winter Squash
- Yellow Squash
- Yucca Root

- Zucchini

Fruits

- Apples NO SEEDS
- Apricots NO PITS
- Bananas & peels
- Bitter Melon
- lack Currants
- Blackberries
- Blueberries
- Boysenberries
- Breadfruit
- Cactus Pear
- Cantaloupe
- Cape Gooseberries
- Cherimoya
- Cherries NO PITS
- Clementines
- Coconut
- Crab Apples
- Cranberries fresh or dried
- Dates
- Durian
- Elderberries – Blue
- Elderberries – Purple Feijoa
- Figs
- Grapefruit

- Grapes, cut in half or quarter to prevent choking
- Uava
- Honeydew Melon
- Huckleberries
- Jackfruit
- Jujube
- Kiwi & peels
- Kumquats
- Lemons
- Limes
- Loganberries
- Lychee
- Mango
- Mulberries
- Nectarine NO PITS
- Olallie berries
- Oranges
- Papayas
- Passion Fruit
- Peaches NO PITS
- Pears NO PITS
- Persimmons
- Pineapple
- Plums NO PITS
- Pomegranate
- Pummelo

- Quince
- Raspberries
- Red Banana
- Red Currants
- Sapodillas
- Sharon Fruit
- Star fruit
- Strawberries
- Tangerines
- Thimbleberry
- Watermelon & rind

GRAINS

- Amaranth
- Barley
- Buckwheat
- Brown Rice, cooked
- Corn
- Farro
- Freekah
- Millet
- Oats / Oatmeal
- Quinoa
- Rye
- Sorghum / Milo
- Teff
- Wheat Varieties:

(spelt, emmer, faro, einkorn, durum, bulgur, cracked wheat, wheat berries)

NUTS & SEEDS (UNSALTED)

- Almonds
- Cashews
- Chia Seeds
- Cumin Seeds
- Brazil Nuts
- BOSS- Black Oil Sunflower Seeds
- Flax Seeds (in moderation)
- Grape Seeds
- Hazelnuts
- Hemp Hearts / Hemp Seeds
- Macadamia Nuts
- Papaya Seeds
- Peanuts
- Pecans
- Pine Nuts
- Pistachios
- Pomegranate Seeds
- Pumpkin Seeds
- Quinoa
- Sesame Seeds
- Sunflower Seeds
- Walnuts
- Wheat Germ

LEGUMES

- Must be cooked – NO canned beans
- Alfalfa
- Black Beans
- Black Eyed Peas
- Boston Beans
- Chick Peas
- Fava Beans
- Field Peas
- Kidney Beans
- Lentils
- Lima Beans
- Mayocoba Beans
- Mung Beans
- Navy Beans
- Pinto Beans
- Red Beans
- Split Peas

SNACKS FOR TREAT DESPENSING TOY

- Any assortment of nuts or seeds
- Oatmeal, plain & dry
- Black Oil Sunflower Seeds
- Raisins
- Dried Cranberries
- Wholegrain Cereals

- (Cheerios, Puffed Rice, Shredded Wheat, Bran Flakes)

SPECIAL SNACKS

- Applesauce, no sugar added
- Baby Food with no sugar or salt added
- Baked cookies or muffins
- (Recipes included)
- Fruit Chips – Bananas, Apples
- Coconut Oil
- Coconut Water
- Cottage Cheese
- Fruit Juice with no sugar added
- Gerber Toddler Puffs
- Granola
- Peanut Butter on celery
- Popcorn Air Popped
- (No oils, butter, or seasoning)
- 100% Pumpkin Canned
- Scrambled or hardboiled eggs
- Warmed/cooked oatmeal
- Whole eggs raw
- Whole Pumpkin
- Yogurt, Plain or Greek

TOXIC FOODS AND PLANTS

- Salt
- Acorns & oak leaves

- Moldy walnut shells
- Elderberries, red berries
- Lima beans, raw
- Kidney beans, raw
- Decayed sweet potatoes (black parts)
- Castor beans
- Tomato leaves and vine
- Avocado – Skin and pit
- Corn stalks (high in nitrates)
- Rhubarb – Leaves (stalk is safe to eat)
- Potato leaves and green parts of potato
- Apple – Leaves & seeds
- Apricot – Leaves & seeds
- Pear – Leaves & seeds
- Peach – Leaves & seeds
- Nectarine – Leaves & seeds
- Cherry – Leaves & seeds
- Plum – Leaves & seeds
- Broccoli – Roots & seeds
- Cabbage – Roots & seeds
- Mustard – Roots & seeds
- Tobacco – leaves
- Nutmeg- in large quantities
- Lychee – seeds

- Rambutan – raw seeds
- Longan – seeds
- Taro – raw
- Cassava roots and leaves
- Almond – Leaves & seeds
  (Only wild or bitter almonds pose a threat, the almonds in stores have been heat treated to eliminate toxicity)
- Raw cashews
  (The cashews at the store are not raw, and are ok to eat)

PLANTS THAT MAY CAUSE PHOTOSENSITIVITY

- Bishop's Weed
- Parsnip tops
- Parsley
- Celery tops
- Giant Hog weed
- Buckwheat
- Saint John 's Wort

CHAPTER 4

BODY CONDITION CHART

SCORE	LAST RIB/ FAT DEPTH (MM)	CONDITION	BODY SHAPE
1	<15	Emaciated	Hips, spine predominant to the eye
2	15-18	Thin	Hips, spine easily felt without pressure
3	18-20	Ideal	Hips, spine felt only with firm pressure
4	20-23	Fat	Hips, spine can not be felt
5	>23	Obese	Hips, spine heavily fat covered

CHAPTER 5

NATURAL DIET GUIDE

All these foods & recipes can be used as healthy snacks within any well balanced diet. If you choose to replace pellets with a natural diet you need to make sure you are meeting all the nutritional requirements of your pig. The best way to do this is variety. The more variety they have in their diet the more opportunity they have to fill all their nutritional needs. Please see "Vitamins and Supplements" on the American Mini Pig Association website for the doses and options.

While pigs thrive on a natural wholesome diet, it's not easy for all pig parents to provide. It can be time consuming and difficult to provide a balanced diet to pigs -- and if a strong commitment to feeding a nutritionally balance varietal diet is not possible, a pelleted diet is best.

In a natural diet plan, the goal is to feed as close as feasible to the variety and nutrients pigs would find in the wild. However, because they aren't in their natural environment, able to forage in different areas and find all the assortment of foods they would naturally come across, it is appropriate to add supplements to make sure they are getting the nutrients that could be missing with grocery store foods.

The same basic principles of mini pig nutrition apply whether they are on a commercial pelleted diet or natural diet. Strive for 12-16 percent protein levels, high fiber, low fat, and as much variety as possible. The bulk of a mini pig's diet should be vegetables. Fruits may be fed on occasion as a treat. Additional elements are: grains, seeds and nuts, beans and lentils, and other healthy foods. Dairy is fine, but should be limited. Meat is fine (unless prohibited by your government) as pigs are omnivores and will consume meat on their own. Avoid pork products that could pose disease risk.

BASIC DAILY DIET:

Each day the pig should get 2 to 3 meals. Vegetables may be given once a day, or with every meal. Grains should be fed once or twice a day. Nuts and seeds should be fed at least once a day. Meat and fish are optional, but may be given as a protein source. Other sources of protein are eggs, lentils, and beans.

Vegetables will make the bulk of the diet. There is no need to limit quantities of vegetables. At minimum they should get a heaping salad at lunch. The more vegetables you can provide, the more satisfied they will be. Vegetables provide essential water content, vitamins, nutrients, and fiber for the gut. Variety is essential for their health, since vegetables are chock full of nutrients, and they all have different nutrient profiles. Dark leafy greens should be fed every day plus a variety of other textures, colors, types. Such as spinach, butternut squash, green beans, banana peels, eggplant, celery, cucumber, and a cherry tomato would be a great day's salad. For a complete list of healthy vegetables please visit the American Mini Pig Association website.

Healthy grains should be given on a daily basis. Wheat bran are the husks of wheat and should be avoided in a mini pig's diet. The bran is high in phosphorus and can cause a calcium-phosphorus imbalance. Grains vary in nutritional values, but tend to stay around 10% protein. Be aware of the protein content to add additional protein into the diet as needed. Grain choices include but are not limited to: amaranth, oats/oatmeal, barley, sorghum/milo, freekah, millet, wheat, wheat berries, wheat germ, spelt, farro, barley, rye, bulgar, teff, and brown rice, quinoa. Rice should always be cooked. Other grains can be given raw, soaked, sprouted, or cooked.

There seems to be consensus that the grains portion of the natural diet should mimic the pellet guide, approx 1/2 cup per day for every 25 lbs body weight split into two meals, then adjust amounts to ensure your pig is maintaining the correct weight. Therefore a pig up to 25 lbs would get 1/4 cup grains in the morning and 1/4 cup at night, plus a hearty mid day salad. A 100 pound pig would get 1 cup of grains in the morning and 1 cup of grains at night. There are many factors that contribute to serving sizes, including age, body condition, and amount of grazing. If your pig is grazing, they will need far less grains.

Seeds and nuts should be incorporated into the daily diet. For the most part, nuts should be shelled. Pieces of shell can get caught in the throats or cause obstruction. These foods provide many essential nutrients, vitamins, and minerals. Many seeds and nuts are high in vitamin e and selenium. They tend to be a nutrition and calorie dense, fatty food. These are healthy calories and healthy fats, but it is wise to feed nuts and seeds in moderation. Add a small portion to a meal (grains or salad), toss them in the yard for the pigs to forage, put them in a treat ball to roll around, or use as training treats and give them a nut/seed for each reward. Nuts and seeds are powerhouse foods, absolutely packed with nutrition. As always, variety is best, as much variety as you can find. However, the basic essentials would be unsalted raw almonds and black oil sunflower seeds. Seeds and nuts should always be unsalted. Healthy choices include but are not limited to: almonds, cashews, brazil nuts, hazelnuts, peanuts, pecans, walnuts, shelled sunflower seeds, black oil sunflower seeds, hemp hearts/hemp seeds, pumpkin seeds, chia seeds, sesame seeds, pomegranate seeds, cumin seeds, grape seeds, papaya seeds.

Lentils and beans are an excellent source of protein and other essential nutrients. These do not need to be fed on a daily basis. Several times a week is sufficient. Lentils and beans should always be cooked or sprouted. Never feed raw beans or lentils to your pig. Avoid canned beans as they can have significantly higher sodium levels. Beans and lentils can be cooked in large batches and frozen into serving sizes for convenience. Beans and lentils provide excellent nutrition, lots of benefits and high in fiber. These powerhouse foods fill many nutritional requirements for the pigs (such as protein, fiber, vitamins, minerals, antioxidants, b vitamins, calcium, potassium, folate, iron). No one bean is perfect as they all have different nutritional makeups. A variety is best. A handful with a salad or as a special side dish would be a great filler. Options include but are not limited to: green lentils, brown lentils, red lentils, azuk, anazazi, black turtle, black eye peas, garbanzo/chickpeas, kidney beans, lima beans, mung beans, navy beans, split peas, cranberry beans, white beans, pinto beans, soybeans, lupin beans, great northern beans, fava beans, cowpeas, and pink beans.

Other foods come in handy for special treats, sick pigs, dispensing medications, and to round out the nutritional balance in your mini pig's meals. Healthy choices include but are not limited to: yogurt, applesauce with no sugar added, canned pumpkin, wholegrain cereals, coconut water, cottage cheese, eggs (raw or cooked, with or without shell), fruit juice with no sugar added, granola, popcorn- air popped from kernels with no salt or oils, peanut butter, raisins.

Mini pigs need a relatively large amount of fiber in their diet. Without sufficient fiber, their gut mobility will slow down increasing the risk of an impaction in the digestive tract. Many pig health problems occur due to too little fiber in the diet. If in doubt, add more fiber! Canned pumpkin, grazing, and dark leafy vegetables are excellent fiber sources.

Pigs are prone to choking and intestinal obstruction, especially with ping pong sized foods. To minimize this risk, chop foods into smaller pieces and cut round foods such as grapes into halves.

CHAPTER 6

SPROUTING FODDER GUIDE

Sprouting fodder for your mini pigs is healthy and simple! Sprouting grains and seeds unleashes the full potential by opening the bioavailability of nutrients. The process of sprouting reduces anti-nutrients in the grain, creating a more digestible food.

Growth of the sprouts is dependent on water and temperature, light isn't required at this stage or growth. Ideal temperatures are 65 to 75 degrees. Sprouting containers can be as large or small as choose, inside or outside, in the bathtub or next to the sink. The only requirement is having an area that you can water and drain completely several times a day.

Seeds and grains must be whole and intact. Dehulled or cracked grains or seeds are not viable for sprouting. Grains and seeds should be untreated (no pesticides or fertilizers). For continual harvest, start a new batch every night. Setup a wire or wooden shelf system to hold trays.

Be sure to take extra care against mold when growing fodder. Moist seeds are a perfect environment for mold to grow, which can be deadly for your pig. NEVER feed a pig molded food, molded seeds, or molded sprouts. Throw any spoiled or molded seeds or grains and start fresh with clean containers.

Step 1:

Place seeds in bucket, cover with plenty of water ensuring room for seeds or grains to expand. Soak seeds or grains in bucket for 8 to 12 hours or overnight.

Step 2:

Pour seeds into shallow plastic container with drain holes along bottom and rinse well. Seeds should be no deeper than ½ inch to avoid mold. Holes need to be small enough to prevent seeds from falling through, but plenty of holes to keep water completely drained. Standing water will drown the seeds/grains and ruin the sprouting process. Ensure good drainage!

Step 3:

Water seeds or grains 2 to 4 times per day, ensuring the water drains promptly. Continue watering daily until sprouts have reached the growth desired. Approximately 5-7 days.

Step 4:

Harvest sprouts or fodder! You can harvest anytime you choose. Sprouted seeds have great nutritional values. As the sprouts grow, they will create a thick root mat and grow greens. After around a week the nutritional needs of the plant will change and it will start to deteriorate if not planted. Feed to mini pigs as a meal or as treats.

Seeds and grains appropriate for sprouting include but are not limited to:

Wheat	Kamut
Barley	Millet
Oats	Quinoa
Black Oil Sunflower Seeds	Rye berries
Amaranth	Sorghum/Milo
Buckwheat	Spelt
Corn	Legumes
Farro	Sesame Seeds

CHAPTER 7

VITAMINS & SUPPLEMENTS GUIDE

Appropriate vitamins and supplements for pigs will vary for each pig, his/her health, dietary needs, environment, age, weight, and feed. There are no hard and fast rules of vitamins or supplements. A high quality, fresh, commercial mini pig pelleted feed is supposed to have everything your pig needs. However, some vitamins and minerals are less stable than others, are damaged during manufacture, improper storage, heat, moisture, or during shelf life. For this reason, some may choose to supplement their pig's diet to ensure they are getting everything they need. When feeding a natural diet, supplements and vitamins may be used to ensure the pigs are getting all the nutrients they require. Supplements and vitamins should be discussed with your veterinarian if you have questions about your pig's individual needs.

The following are optional supplements pig owners may choose for their pigs. You do not need to use all supplements listed. Remember that oils are lubricating and will lubricate the digestive tract if introduced too fast. Start slow with oils and increase dosage to bowel tolerance. Also keep in mind calories. Oils are calorie dense. Fed in excess, or in a diet of other excess, oils can contribute to obesity. Supplements are not "free" calories just because they are healthy. Consider your pig's overall food and nutritional intake when adding supplements. Some vitamins, minerals, or supplements are toxic if overdosed, others will be excreted in urine if not needed.

Two supplements that are recommended for all pet pigs are selenium and vitamin e. Although commercial feeds are formulated with these nutrients, the vitamin e and selenium availability after manufacture and storage is variable. A deficiency in either of these nutrients may cause debilitating disease or sudden death.

VITAMIN E: (HIGHLY RECOMMENDED)

Vitamin E is one of the most important additions to your pig's diet. It is an essential nutrient in the body and works with selenium to keep the pig healthy. A deficiency in either of these will result in a painful and possibly lethal disease. There are many factors that influence vitamin E concentrations and requirements. Some of these include: artificial drying of grains, storage time and conditions, unsaturated fatty acids, and selenium concentrations. Vitamin E, even though added to commercial mini pig pellets, will break down with improper storage, during manufacture of feed, and during a normal shelf life. Due to the importance of this vitamin in the body and the instability of the vitamin in commercial feeds, the only way to ensure your pig is getting enough is to supplement.

One 400 IU capsule per day will provide sufficient vitamin E for your pig with no toxic risks.

Foods naturally rich in Vitamin E: almonds, raw sunflower seeds, pumpkin seeds, sesame seeds, swiss chard, mustard greens, spinach, turnip greens, kale, plant oils, hazelnuts, pine nuts, broccoli, and papaya.

SELENIUM: (HIGHLY RECOMMENDED)

Selenium is an essential nutrient. It is added to good quality mini pig feed pellets. Cathy Corrigan DVM has advised an additional selenium dose of 150 to 300 mcg given ONCE PER WEEK. You will find selenium supplements in the human supplement aisle at the store. Alternately, may use a horse vitamin e/selenium supplements from Tractor Supply or your local farm store. ElevateSe is a good horse supplement you can give to your pigs instead of the human selenium tablet. ElevateSe can be given at the dose of 1 tsp each week.

Many healthy foods are good sources of selenium but the actual selenium levels in the foods vary depending on the selenium content of the soil it was grown in. Some parts of the United States have selenium deficient soil, producing selenium deficient crops. It is safest to add once a week supplement to avoid terrible and devastating nutritional deficiencies. However, selenium is toxic if overdosed. Only a small amount is needed, be careful to not overdose. Mini pigs fed a commercial diet should not be given selenium supplementation more than once per week.

Foods naturally rich in selenium include: barley, brown rice, sunflower seeds, flaxseeds, cabbage, spinach, broccoli, swiss chard, whole grains, nuts, and seeds.

MULTIVITAMIN:

Most pigs may benefit from a good quality children's multivitamin daily. Young piglets can have 1/2 children's vitamin daily. Pigs over 6 months or 25 lbs can have 1 children's vitamin daily. Be aware gummy vitamins are terrible for dental health, as any chewy foods are, and loaded with sugar. Some pig owners prefer to find a vitamin with no aspartame (artificial sweetener) or gelatin (often includes porcine ingredients).

YUCCA ROOT:

Yucca root is an extraordinary supplement useful for a variety of reasons. This supplement is truly one of nature's miracles. However, it can cause problems if given in large quantity. Supplement in moderation, only as needed. Always consult your veterinarian with any questions, concerns, or recommendations.

Benefits may include:

- pain relief
- anti inflammatory
- decreases feces odors
- aids in digestion
- appetite stimulant for weak or ill pigs
- relieve skin issues when used in shampoos

- vitamin C, beta-carotene, calcium, iron, manganese, magnesium, niacin, phosphorous, protein, and B vitamins

According to Clara Fenger, DVM, PhD, DACVIM, the dose recommendation for decreasing the ammonia in the feces is about one teaspoon per day.

Use 100% pure Yucca Schidigera root.

COCONUT OIL:

Coconut oil is a great supplement for pigs. You can pour it over their food, rub it on them, or refrigerate it into bite sized treats using a mini muffin pan, silicone mold, or ice cube tray. 1 tablespoon per 25 pounds daily. Coconut oil is great for skin and hair health among other benefits. Order the AMPA Mini Pig Cookbook from the American Mini Pig Store or check out the AMPA Blog Recipes for great coconut oil treat recipes!

REFINED OR UNREFINED?

Refined or unrefined coconut oil is a personal preference. Either variety is ok, but they are distinctly different. Unrefined has purity and added health benefits. Organic Virgin Cold Pressed coconut oil is going to have the most nutrients and health benefits.

Unrefined coconut oil may be referred to as virgin or pure. This is the preferred form of coconut oil for nutritional supplementation and health benefits. Processing the fresh coconut meat prevents contamination found in other methods, so the harsh chemicals used for refined coconut oil aren't needed. Unrefined coconut oil has more phytonutrients and polyphenols. Unrefined coconut oil is richer in proteins, vitamins, and anti oxidants. This variety of coconut oil smells and tastes of fresh coconut. If you choose unrefined, organic is best, look for "pure" "unrefined" "virgin" or "extra virgin" "cold pressed" on the label. Unrefined coconut oil can be processed as Cold Pressed or Expeller Pressed. Cold pressing retains more nutrients than expeller pressed.

Refined coconut oil has been through a manufacturing process. This manufacturing process may use bleach or other harsh chemicals. These chemicals will not be on the label because they are used in processing, not an ingredient. Food regulations only require ingredients on the label. The reason to use bleach and harsh chemicals is to whiten the oil, to deodorize to remove the distinct coconut scent and flavor, and added sodium hydroxide to prolong its shelf life. Many nutritive factors are damaged or destroyed during the refinement process such as phytonutrients. Refined coconut oil is typically derived from coconut meat that has been dried (copra). The benefits of refined coconut oil are cost, absent flavor (good for baking), and a higher smoking point of 450 degrees (unrefined coconut oil has a smoking point of 350 degrees).

Cold Pressed or Expeller pressed

Cold pressed coconut oil is processed at or below 120 degrees. It will have a mild coconut flavor. This lower temperature processing preserves more nutrients than other methods, particularly the phenolic compounds.

Expeller pressed coconut oil is processed at higher temperatures resulting in a more toasted coconut flavor. This method uses a higher temperature than cold pressed, losing some nutrients int he process. This is still far lower temperature than refined coconut oil, therefore preserves more of the nutrients.

Benefits of coconut oil internally (eaten)

- Vitamin E, Vitamin K, and iron
- Lauric acic, CAprylic acid, and Capric acid
- Antiviral
- Antibacterial
- Antiyeast
- Antifungal
- Anticanver
- Boosts immune system
- Supports healthy skin
- Promotes heart health
- Promotes healthy brain function
- Supports thyroid function
- Promotes healthy skin
- Has been shown to dramatically reduce seizures in epileptic children
- Benefits of coconut oil externally
- Moisturizes dry skin
- Promotes healthy hair
- Heals cracks and chapped skin
- Heals minor sunburn (avoid sun!)
- Antiviral
- Antibacterial
- Helps to sooth and heal damaged irritated skin
- Scratches
- Bug bites
- Used on teeth promotes dental health

FISH OIL:

Healthy pigs can be given 100 to 150 mg EPA and DHA per 10 pounds of body weight daily; pigs who have health problems (arthritis, seasonal allergies, or dry skin) can be given up to 300 mg per 10 pounds of body weight.

With fish oil, check the ingredients. You want as few ingredients as possible. Gelatin and glycerin are common to make the capsule. No getting around that. Tocopherols are used as a preservative and stabilizer. No problem. Avoid anything extra, you don't want rosemary or anything else added. Look for "fish oil" not enteric coated or burpless, just fish oil.

Fish oil is one of the most commonly used supplements in veterinary medicine. It is so well known and used that it is considered a mainstream or conventional medication instead of an alternative medication. This has the benefit of bringing a lot of exposure and clinical experience of fish oil use in pets. Fish oil supports their heart health and immune system

With fish oil you want to look at the total Omega-3. On the back will show DHA, EPA, and Total OMEGA-3. It's the total Omega 3 you look at for dosing. Also check the serving size. That # can be for 1 capsule or 2 capsules. Introduce any oil into your pig's diet slowly or you will deal with diarrhea while their digestive tracts adjust. Most pills are 300 to 360 Omega-3 per pill. If it says 720 Omega-3, check serving size, that may be for 2 pills, meaning each pill would be 360 mg. You can also find more concentrated fish oil pills with a higher concentration of Omega-3 requiring less pills per day for larger pigs.

Benefits may include:

- Nourishes & promotes healthy skin and hair
- Reduces inflammation
- Reduces arthritis pain
- Boost in immune system
- Aids in fighting infections
- Reduced joint discomfort
- Increased stamina
- Reduced risk of stroke or heart problems
- Antioxidant properties lower cancer risk
- Relief of allergy symptoms
- Helpful in treating kidney disease
- May shrink tumors

IRON:

Adult or mature pigs do not need supplemental iron. These pigs have a very low need for iron and excess iron can be toxic. They are able to get iron from rooting in the dirt. If they have no access to the outdoors it's best to feed them iron rich foods. Young piglets with no access to dirt may be given a 1/2 children's vitamin with iron 2-3 times per week. A better solution would be to bring in some dirt for them to root through daily to get a variety of essential minerals.

According to Cathy Corrigan DVM, too much iron supplementation "can select for bad enteric bacteria and cause significant diarrhea. Enough is in the pelleted diets and things like spinach that she does not need to worry about it. Iron supplementation is for young piglets, those with whip worms, and those that have bleeding for some reason."

Foods naturally rich in iron include: spinach, other dark leafy greens, beans (lima beans, red kidney beans, chickpeas, or split peas), lentils, breakfast cereals enriched with iron, wheat germ, rice, sunflower seeds and nuts (peanuts, pecans, walnuts, pistachios, almonds, cashews).

BIOTIN:

Biotin is a coenzyme and a B vitamin, an essential nutrient that is used for hair, skin and nail (hoof) growth. It is available in many natural foods and also in pig pelleted feed. Some pigs may require extra biotin. If your pigs hair or hooves are dry, brittle, sparse, or cracking, then a biotin supplement may help the pig with new healthier growth (of hair and hooves). 1 biotin supplement daily per pig. These will come in capsule or gummy forms in the human supplement aisle. 1,000 mcg biotin daily is sufficient for the needs of most mini pigs.

Or, you can give Horseshoers Secret which is a horse pelleted supplement. It supplies biotin, zinc, trace minerals, and omega fatty acids to help with healthy skin and hooves. 1 teaspoon per week is recommended for pigs.

Foods naturally rich in biotin include nuts, root vegetables, and eggs.

VITAMIN C:

For healthy skin. If a pig is taking a multi-vitamin there is no need for extra Vitamin C. If skin conditions persist, supplemental Vitamin C may improve skin condition if the condition is due to a deficiency of Vitamin C. You can find pills or gummy vitamins in the pharmacy. Dose is 500 mg daily per pig.

WHEAT GERM OIL:

Wheat Germ Oil is another supplement that some use internally or externally. Oral dose is 1 ounce daily mixed with food. Store in fridge to prevent oil from going rancid. Can also be used in cooking/baking treats or mixed in with pellets, yogurt, or pumpkin.

Benefits internally:

- Promotes skin & hair health
- Rich in Vitamin E
- Rich in essential fatty acids Omega 3-6-9
- Rich in magnesium
- Rich in vitamin B, helps repair tissues
- Promotes stable blood sugar levels

APPLE CIDER VINEGAR:

Said to be beneficial in many ways, although little has been proven. Can be used internally or externally. Available at the grocery store. Unfiltered, organic or raw apple cider vinegar is preferred for the health benefits. Also offer plain water in a separate bowl nearby in case your pet chooses not to drink the ACV to prevent dehydration.

Benefits of ACV may include:

- Supports natural body functions Supports healthy urinary tract
- Relief of constipation
- Supports immune system

- Promotes digestion and ph balance
- Supports healthy skin
- Supports healthy gut bacteria
- High in potassium
- Stabilizes blood sugar levels
- Soothes sunburn, insect bites, abrasions, stings, and other skin ailments
- Insect repellent
- Increases absorption of essential nutrients in other foods
- Scours, or loose stool

DIATOMACEOUS EARTH:

Not exactly a supplement, but used as a chemical free natural dewormer when fed to pigs (ONLY FOOD GRADE DE) to rid them of intestinal parasites. This has not been proven effective and many pigs that are dewormed with DE will be full of roundworms. When used in conjunction with chemical dewormers such as ivermectin and fenbendazole you'll be sure to have all bases covered.

Also can be applied to their skin to rid them of fleas, although it is very drying and will exacerbate dry skin. Can be sprinkled on their beds, blankets, indoors, outdoors, in the yard, on the dirt, all over their environment to eradicate many pests. Sprinkle over poop to control flies and other insects.

Since it is safe to eat it's totally find to sprinkle where they graze. Also safe for dogs and other pets. Can be found at Tractor Supply or other farm stores. Must be food grade. It's so safe and natural that many people ingest it also.

CANNED PUMPKIN:

Not a supplement, but very useful none the less. 100% pure pumpkin. It will bulk and binds food together so will help relieve constipation and diarrhea. This is not pumpkin pie filling even though there is a picture of pumpkin pie on the front. Look for "100% pure" and on the back look at ingredients. The only ingredient should be pumpkin. Great as a snack and for sneaking in liquid medications also. Mix worming medications or other liquids into the pumpkin for a special snack and they won't even know they took their medications. Should be fed to pigs as surgery care to keep their bowels moving. Anesthesia and pain medications are constipating, pain will further the constipation causing them to not eat and complications may develop including ulcers. 1/4 can of pumpkin twice a day before and after surgery will keep everything moving as it should.

CHAPTER 8

DRINKS

Hydration is important for maintaining a healthy body. Water intake helps with food digestion and elimination, blood circulation, it helps nutrients flow, and it keeps our pig's cool on hot days. Adding tasty variations of juices, or infusing fruits and herbs can help encourage good water intake.

ACV Health Boosting Splash

Ingredients:

1 cup unrefined apple cider vinegar "with the mother"

1 gallon fresh water

Instructions:

Combine water and ACV. Unrefined apple cider vinegar is touted as a hugely beneficial supplement for overall health. Word of caution: some pigs may find the taste unpleasant and will avoid drinking. Be sure to keep a separate bowl of fresh plain water to encourage hydration.

Coconut Cucumber Cooler

Ingredients:

1 cup coconut water

1 cucumber, sliced

1 gallon water

Instructions:

Combine all ingredients in water dish.

Cranberry Coconut Refresher

Ingredients:

1 part cranberry juice

1 part coconut water

4 parts water

Instructions:

Pour ingredients in drinking bowl. Enjoy fresh!

Daily Dose of Cranberry

½ cup cranberry juice

1 gallon water

Instructions:

Combine ingredients in water dish.

Apple Cranberry UTI Buster

Ingredients:

½ cup unrefined apple cider vinegar

½ cup cranberry juice

¼ cup diced apples

¼ cup cranberries, fresh or frozen

1 gallon water

Instructions:

Mix all ingredients in water dish.

Sick Pig Saver

Ingredients:

½ cup low sodium broth

1 cup water

Instructions:

Combine ingredients, warm slightly. Offer to pig in water dish, bowl, or syringe drops slowly into the mouth, making sure they are swallowing. This can be used to entice sick or dehydrated pigs to drink, helping them to gain strength and appetite.

Infused Water – Multiple Varieties!

Choose ingredients from below, or create your own variety with herbs, spices, edible flowers, fruits and vegetables. Place ingredients into bottle, mason jar, or pitcher. If using ice, add ice to container. Fill with water and refrigerate overnight.

Enjoy fresh as drinking water with a snack, or freeze into ice cube trays for use in water bowls. Excellent for encouraging healthy hydration! Infused water provides essential vitamins and nutrients without unnecessary calories or artificial sweeteners. Plus, it tastes great! Fruit infused water has less calories, less sugar, and better flavor than grocery store juices. Extend the flavor of fruits in your pig's diet.

TIPS: Do not use bruised or wilted foods. Chop or slice foods into smaller pieces for more flavorful water. Optional, a muddler can be used to crush foods before ice and/or water is added. Use or freeze within 3 days. Add in coconut water, unrefined apple cider vinegar, cranberry juice, or chia seeds to any recipe for additional health benefits. Use citrus sparingly for just a hint of flavor without excess acidity.

Blueberry Mint Lemonade Infused Water

Ingredients: blueberries, lemon slices, mint leaves

Basil Citrus Infused Water

Instructions: basil, orange slices

Raspberry Apple Infused Water

Ingredients: apple slices, raspberries, rosemary

Minty Cucumber Pineapple Infused Water

Ingredients: mint leaves, cucumber slices, pineapple chunks

Blackberry Kiwi Infused Water

Ingredients: blackberries, kiwi slices

Strawberry Basil Infused Water

Ingredients: strawberry slices, basil

Strawberry Kiwi Lime Infused Water

Ingredients: strawberry slices, lime slices, kiwi slices

Lemon Lime Infused Water

Ingredients: lemon slices, lime slices

Pina Colada Infused Water

Ingredients: pineapple chunks, coconut chunks

Raspberry Mint Infused Water

Ingredients: raspberries, mint leaves

Orange Blueberry Infused Water

Ingredients: orange slices, blueberries

Melon Basil Infused Water

Ingredients: watermelon, basil leaves

Cucumber Mint Infused Water

Ingredients: cucumber slices, mint

Blue Kiwi Infused Water

Ingredients: blueberry, kiwi slices

Blackberry Cherry Limeade Infused Water

Ingredients: blackberries, cherries, lime slices

Lemon Cucumber Mint Infused Water

Ingredients: lemon slices, cucumber slices, mint leaves

Lemon Raspberry Mint Infused Water

Ingredients: lemon slices, raspberries, mint leaves

Blueberry Lime Infused Water

Ingredients: blueberry, lime

Minty Melon Infused Water

Ingredients: watermelon, honeydew melon, mint leaves

Blueberry Pineapple Infused Water

Ingredients: Blueberries, pineapple

Summer Burst Infused Water

Ingredients: strawberries, orange slices, blueberries

Mango Lime Basil Infused Water

Ingredients: mango, lime slices, basil leaves

Raspberry Ginger Basil Infused Water

Ingredients: raspberries, ginger, basil

Strawberry Melon Minty Infused Water

Ingredients: strawberry slices, watermelon, mint leaves

Lemon Berry Infused Water

Ingredients: lemon slices, raspberries, blueberries

Kiwi Raspberry Mint Infused Water

Ingredients: kiwi, raspberry, mint leaves

Sweet Fruit Nectar Infused Water

Ingredients: peach, honey dew, cantaloupe

Cinnamon Apple Infused Water

Ingredients: apple slices, cinnamon stick

Triple Berry Sage Infused Water

Ingredients: raspberries, blueberries, strawberries, sage

Watermelon Peach Infused Water

Ingredients: watermelon, peach

Pineapple Mint Infused Water

Ingredients: pineapple, mint leaves

Blackberry Sage Infused Water

Ingredients: blackberries, sage

Watermelon Rosemary Infused Water

Ingredients: watermelon, rosemary

Minty Melon Infused Water

Ingredients: watermelon, mint leaves

Strawberry Orange Infused Water

Ingredients: strawberries, orange slices

Strawberry Limeade Infused Water

Ingredients: strawberries, lemon slices, lime slices

Orange Raspberry Rosemary Infused Water

Ingredients: orange slices, raspberries, rosemary

Blueberry Lavender Infused Water

Ingredients: blueberries, lavender flowers or leaves

Refreshing Detox Infused Water

Ingredients: orange slices, cucumber slices, mint leaves

Cinnamon Pear Ginger Infused Water

Ingredients: cinnamon stick, pear slices, grated ginger

Mango Ginger Infused Water

Ingredients: mango, grated ginger

Raspberry Orange Infused Water

Ingredients: raspberries, orange slices

Coconut Cucumber Infused Water

Ingredients: coconut water, cucumber slices

Peach Mint Infused Water

Ingredients: peach slices, mint leaves

CHAPTER 9

SMOOTHIES AND FROZEN DRINKS

Green Power Smoothie

Ingredients:

½ cup frozen mango cubes

½ cup chopped cucumber

1 cup baby spinach

2 tbsp fresh mint leaves

½ cup coconut water

Instructions:

Pour all ingredients into blender. Puree until smooth. Serve fresh.

Pumpkin Smoothie

Ingredients:

½ cup canned pumpkin

½ frozen fruit (peaches, mango, etc)

½ cup almond milk

½ cup coconut water

Instructions:

In blender, puree all ingredients. Serve fresh or freeze into silicone mold or ice cube trays for individual frozen treats.

Coconut Pumpkin Smoothie

Ingredients:

1 cup ice

½ cup coconut water

¾ cup canned pumpkin

Instructions:

Blend all ingredients in blender until smooth. Serve fresh or freeze into silicone mold or ice cube trays for individual frozen treats.

Berries & Beets Smoothie

Ingredients:

½ cup blueberries

½ cup raspberries

½ cup sliced, cooked beets

¼ cup yogurt

¼ cup coconut water

Instructions:

Blend all ingredients in blender until smooth. Serve fresh or freeze into silicone mold or ice cube trays for individual frozen treats.

Berry Oat Smoothie

Ingredients:

¼ cup oatmeal, cooked

¼ cup unsweetened almond milk

1 cup mixed berries

½ cup strawberries

1 tbsp wheat germ

½ cup ice (optional)

Instructions:

Blend all ingredients in blender until smooth. Serve fresh or freeze into silicone mold or ice cube trays for individual frozen treats.

Almond Spinach Smoothie

Ingredients:

½ cup fresh spinach

¾ cup unsweetened almond milk

1 frozen banana

1 tbsp almond butter

1 tbsp wheat germ

Instructions:

Blend all ingredients in blender until smooth. Serve fresh or freeze into silicone mold or ice cube trays for individual frozen treats.

Cool Mint Smoothie

Ingredients:

1 cucumber

1 small beet

¼ cup pineapple, frozen

Mint leaves

Instructions:

Blend all ingredients in blender until smooth. Serve fresh or freeze into silicone mold or ice cube trays for individual frozen treats.

Minty Watermelon Cucumber Smoothie

Ingredients:

1 cup watermelon, frozen chunks

1 cucumber

¼ cup coconut water

1 tbsp chia seeds

Mint leaves

Instructions:

Blend all ingredients in blender until smooth. Serve fresh or freeze into silicone mold or ice cube trays for individual frozen treats.

Blueberry Cucumber Smoothie

Ingredients:

1 cucumber

½ cup plain yogurt

1 cup blueberries

1 tbsp wheat germ

Instructions:

Blend all ingredients in blender until smooth. Serve fresh or freeze into silicone mold or ice cube trays for individual frozen treats.

Hydration Therapy Smoothie

Ingredients:

½ cup plain yogurt

1 cucumber

Mint leaves

½ cup almond milk

Instructions:

Blend all ingredients in blender until smooth. Serve fresh or freeze into silicone mold or ice cube trays for individual frozen treats.

Berry Cool Smoothie

Ingredients:

1 cucumber

½ cup berries, frozen

½ cup mangos, frozen

½ cup almond milk

Instructions:

Blend all ingredients in blender until smooth. Serve fresh or freeze into silicone mold or ice cube trays for individual frozen treats.

Summer Break Smoothie

Ingredients:

1 cucumber

1 cup watermelon, frozen

½ cup cantaloupe, frozen

½ cup coconut water

Instructions:

Blend all ingredients in blender until smooth. Serve fresh or freeze into silicone mold or ice cube trays for individual frozen treats.

Cranberry Pumpkin Smoothie

Ingredients:

1 cup canned pumpkin

½ cup cranberry juice

Instructions:

Blend all ingredients in blender until smooth. Serve fresh or freeze into silicone mold or ice cube trays for individual frozen treats.

Banana Berry Superfood Smoothie

Ingredients

½ cup cranberries

½ cup mixed berries, frozen

1 banana, frozen

1 cup almond or coconut milk

1 tbsp chia seeds

¼ cup rolled oats

Instructions:

Blend all ingredients in blender until smooth. Serve fresh or freeze into silicone mold or ice cube trays for individual frozen treats.

Cranberry Banana Smoothie

Ingredients:

1 cup cranberries, frozen

1 banana, frozen

1 cup almond milk

Instructions:

Blend all ingredients in blender until smooth. Serve fresh or freeze into silicone mold or ice cube trays for individual frozen treats.

Cranberry Orange Smoothie

1 cup cranberries, frozen

½ cup orange juice

½ cup yogurt

¼ cup rolled oats

Instructions:

Blend all ingredients in blender until smooth. Serve fresh or freeze into silicone mold or ice cube trays for individual frozen treats.

Vitamin C Burst Smoothie

Ingredients:

1 orange, peeled

1 cup cranberries, frozen

1 cup peaches, frozen

½ cup almond milk

Instructions:

Blend all ingredients in blender until smooth. Serve fresh or freeze into silicone mold or ice cube trays for individual frozen treats.

Minty Melon Smoothie

Ingredients:

2 cups seedless watermelon

2 tbsp fresh mint

1/3 cup plain yogurt

Instructions:

Blend all ingredients in blender until smooth. Serve fresh or freeze into silicone mold or ice cube trays for individual frozen treats.

Strawberry Coconut Smoothie

Ingredients:

1 cup strawberries, frozen

1 banana, frozen

½ cup unsweetened almond milk

¼ cup shredded unsweetened coconut

½ cup plain yogurt

Instructions:

Blend all ingredients in blender until smooth. Serve fresh or freeze into silicone mold or ice cube trays for individual frozen treats.

Blend all ingredients in blender until smooth. Serve fresh or freeze into silicone mold or ice cube trays for individual frozen treats.

Berry Melon Smoothie

Ingredients:

2 cups seedless watermelon

1 cup strawberries, frozen

Instructions:

Blend all ingredients in blender until smooth. Serve fresh or freeze into silicone mold or ice cube trays for individual frozen treats.

Spring Fever Smoothie

Ingredients:

½ cup coconut milk

1 banana, frozen

½ cup mango, frozen

½ cup strawberries, frozen

1 tbsp chia seeds

Instructions:

Blend all ingredients in blender until smooth. Serve fresh or freeze into silicone mold or ice cube trays for individual frozen treats.

Cooling Cucumber Smoothie

Ingredients:

1 cucumber

½ cup blueberries, frozen

¼ cup coconut water

Instructions:

Berry Green Smoothie

Ingredients:

1 cup spinach, chopped

1 cup water

½ cup blueberries, frozen

½ cup mixed berries, frozen

1 banana

1 kiwi

1 tsp chia seeds

Instructions:

Blend all ingredients in blender until smooth. Serve fresh or freeze into silicone mold or ice cube trays for individual frozen treats.

Peach Coconut Green Smoothie

Ingredients:

1 cup spinach, chopped

½ cup coconut water

1 cup grapes

1 cup peaches, frozen

1 tbsp coconut oil

Instructions:

Blend all ingredients in blender until smooth. Serve fresh or freeze into silicone mold or ice cube trays for individual frozen treats.

Healthy Turned Delish Smoothie

Ingredients:

1 cup spinach, chopped

1 cup almond milk

½ cup sweet potato, cooked

1 cup mango, frozen

1 tbsp flax seeds

Instructions:

Blend all ingredients in blender until smooth. Serve fresh or freeze into silicone mold or ice cube trays for individual frozen treats.

Superfood Smoothie Gone Green

Ingredients:

1 cup spinach, chopped

1 cup almond milk

1 apple, cored

1 banana, frozen

¼ cup rolled oats

2 tbsp coconut oil

1 tbsp brewers yeast

Instructions:

Blend all ingredients in blender until smooth. Serve fresh or freeze into silicone mold or ice cube trays for individual frozen treats.

Cranberry Kale Smoothie

Ingredients:

1 cup fresh kale, chopped

1 cup cranberry juice

1 orange, peeled

1 tsbp chia seeds

1 cup ice (optional)

Instructions:

Blend all ingredients in blender until smooth. Serve fresh or freeze into silicone mold or ice cube trays for individual frozen treats.

Tropical Green Smoothie

Ingredients:

1 cup fresh spinach or kale

½ cup coconut water

½ cup mango, frozen

½ cup pineapple

1 banana, frozen

1 tbsp chia seeds

Instructions:

Blend all ingredients in blender until smooth. Serve fresh or freeze into silicone mold or ice cube trays for individual frozen treats.

Powerhouse Pumpkin Smoothie

Ingredients:

¼ cup chickpeas, cooked

¼ cup oats

½ cup canned pumpkin

½ cup almond milk

2 tbsp chia seeds

Instructions:

Blend all ingredients in blender until smooth. Serve fresh or freeze into silicone mold or ice cube trays for individual frozen treats.

Almond Berry Smoothie

½ cup blueberries, frozen

½ cup strawberries, frozen

½ cup almond milk

1 tbsp wheat germ

Instructions:

Blend all ingredients in blender until smooth. Serve fresh or freeze into silicone mold or ice cube trays for individual frozen treats.

Fall Feast Smoothie

Ingredients:

1 sweet potato, baked & cooled

½ cup cranberries, frozen

½ cup almond milk

1 tsp brewers yeast

Instructions:

Blend all ingredients in blender until smooth. Serve fresh or freeze into silicone mold or ice cube trays for individual frozen treats.

CHAPTER 10

SOUPS

Garden Harvest Soup

Ingredients:

1 cup chopped uncooked vegetables (squash, zucchini, green beans, carrots)

1 cup fresh spinach leaves, coarsely chopped

3-4 cherry tomatoes

¼ cup pumpkin puree

1 cups water

Instructions:

Combine all ingredients except spinach in stovetop sauce pan. Bring to a boil and simmer until vegetables are tender. Remove from heat, stir in spinach, allow to cool, and serve.

Lentil Stew

Ingredients:

1 tbsp olive oil

1 stalk celery diced

1 carrot, diced

½ cup dried lentils

¼ cup pumpkin puree

2 cups water

Instructions:

In soup pot, heat olive oil on medium heat. Sauté celery and carrots for 5 minutes. Stir in lentils and water. Bring to a boil, then reduce to simmer. Cover and simmer for 40 minutes. Then, stir in spinach until it wilts. Remove from heat, allow to cool, and serve.

Pumpkin Soup

Ingredients:

1 cup canned pumpkin

¼ cup low sodium vegetable broth

½ cup coconut milk

Optional:

Raw pumpkin seeds

Oats

Instructions:

Simmer ingredients over medium heat on stove. Allow to cool, top with oats and raw pumpkin seeds.

Quinoa Veggie Soup

Ingredients:

1 carrot, chopped

1 parsnip, chopped

1 celery stalk, chopped

1 cup zucchini or squash, chopped

1 cup quinoa

½ cup diced tomatoes

3 cups water

½ cup canned pumpkin

½ cup cooked chickpeas

¾ cup kale and/or collard greens, chopped

Instructions:

In stove top soup pot, combine water, carrot, parsnip, celery, zucchini, squash, tomatoes, and quinoa. Bring to a boil and simmer for 25 minutes stirring occasionally. Add in chickpeas, kale, collard greens, and canned pumpkin. Simmer for an additional 5-10 minutes. Allow to cool, serve fresh, or separate into portions and freeze for later use.

Butternut Squash Soup Feast

Ingredients:

1 butternut squash, halved

2 carrots, diced

4 cups diced apples

5 cups water

Vegetable oil for sautéing

Instructions:

Preheat oven to 400 degrees. Place butternut squash halves on parchment paper lined baking sheet. Bake for 35 to 45 minutes or until cooked. Meanwhile, sauté carrots and apples in olive oil on stove. Scoop out seeds and set aside to top on a salad or other meal. Scoop squash flesh and put in blender with ¼ cup water. Puree until smooth. Next, puree apples and carrots. Heat remaining water in soup pot. Gently stir in pureed vegetables. Bring to a slow boil and simmer 5 minutes, stirring to mix well. Serve fresh as a hydrating treat. Freeze extra portions for later meals. Especially useful during times of illness, surgery recovery, or dehydration.

Coconut Pea Soup

Ingredients:

1 ½ cups water

½ can coconut milk, or 7 ounces

1 pound frozen green peas

Instructions:

Pour all ingredients in soup pot. Bring to a boil, then simmer 10 minutes. Remove from heat. Puree soup with handheld immersion blender. Serve fresh or freeze individual portions for later meals.

Chickpea Chard Stew

Ingredients:

2 cups water

2 cups diced tomatoes

1 cup chickpeas, cooked

1 bunch of chard, stems removed and leaves cut into strips

¼ cup basil leaves, chopped (optional)

Instructions:

Combine all ingredients in soup pot on stove. Bring to a boil, then simmer 10 minutes. Serve fresh or freeze individual portions for later meals.

Cream of Artichoke Soup

Ingredients:

½ cup frozen cauliflower florets, thawed

2 cups frozen artichoke hearts, thawed

3 cups water

Instructions:

In large soup pot, bring all ingredients to a boil. Simmer 15 minutes. Allow to cool enough to use blender to puree soup. Serve fresh or freeze individual portions for later meals.

Vegetable Soup with Pumpkin Broth

Ingredients:

¼ cup cooked grains/lentils (oats, wheat, barley, brown rice, lentils)

¼ cup chopped vegetables

½ cup warm water

¼ cup canned pumpkin

Instructions:

Combine all ingredients, serve fresh or store in fridge.

Pumpkin Barley Stew

¼ cup cooked barley

½ cup frozen pumpkin chunks, thawed

Handful of frozen pumpkin seeds, thawed

½ cup spinach, chopped

1 cup warm water

2 tbsp black oil sunflower seeds

Instructions:

On stovetop, bring water, barley, pumpkin, and spinach to a simmer until spinach wilts and soup is warm. Remove from heat. Sprinkle pumpkin seeds and black oil sunflower seeds on top. Serve fresh.

CHAPTER 11

SALADS

Classic Kale Salad

Ingredients:

1 cup kale

¼ cup cranberries

3-4 almonds

Instructions:

Combine all ingredients. Serve fresh.

Blueberry Chard Salad

Ingredients:

1 cup swiss chard

¼ cup blueberries

2 tsp chia seeds

Instructions:

Combine all ingredients. Serve fresh.

Green Bean Salad

Ingredients:

1 cup green beans

1 tomato, diced

¼ cup corn, fresh or frozen

Instructions:

Combine all ingredients. Serve fresh.

Cucumber Beet Salad

Ingredients:

1 arugula

½ cup beets, sliced

1 cucumber sliced

Instructions:

Combine all ingredients. Serve fresh.

Salad Bar Gazpacho

Ingredients:

¼ cups chickpeas, red kidney beans, and/or black beans

1/2 cup diced tomatoes, cucumbers, and corn

2 tbsp minced cilantro

1 cup mixed greens

Instructions:

On plate, arrange mixed greens. Cover with remaining ingredients and sprinkle cilantro on top.

Cucumber Salad

Ingredients:

1 cucumber, sliced

1 tbsp melted coconut oil

1 tomato, chopped

1 tbsp sesame seeds

Instructions:

Mix cucumber slices, tomatoes, and coconut oil. Sprinkle sesame seeds on top. Serve fresh.

Kale Quinoa Salad

Ingredients:

1 cup quinoa, cooked

2 cups kale, chopped

¼ cup cranberries, dried or fresh

2 tbsp black oil sunflower seeds

2 tbsp chia seeds

Instructions:

Mix together ingredients. Serve fresh.

Walnut Lentil Salad

Ingredients

½ cup cooked lentils

½ cup diced pumpkin or acorn squash

¼ cup chopped walnuts

2 cups mixed greens

Instructions:

Mix ingredients and serve fresh.

Lentil Squash Salad

Ingredients:

½ cup lentils, cooked

½ cup acorn squash, cubed

¼ cup beets, chopped

½ cup mustard greens, chopped

Instructions:

Combine all ingredients. Serve fresh.

Bountiful Harvest Salad

Ingredients:

½ cup parsnips, chopped

½ cup turnips, chopped

½ cup kale, chopped

½ cup swiss chard, chopped

½ cup collard greens, chopped

¼ cup cranberries

Instructions:

Layer ingredients over.

Cranberry Almond Spinach Salad

Ingredients:

8 oz baby spinach

½ cup sliced almonds

½ cup cranberries, fresh or dried

2 tbs sesame seeds

Instructions:

Layer salad ingredients on a plate. Serve fresh.

Cranberry Broccoli Salad

Ingredients:

1 cup broccoli, diced, cooked or raw

½ cup cranberries, dried or fresh

¼ cup walnuts, chopped

½ apple, sliced

Instructions:

Mix ingredients together. Serve fresh.

Orange Pecan Spinach Salad

Ingredients:

8 ounces baby spinach

1 small can orange segments, drained

¼ cup chopped pecans

¼ cup cranberries, dried or fresh

2 tablespoons coconut oil, melted

1 tablespoon chia seeds

Instructions:

Arrange salad ingredients. Drizzle melted coconut oil on top. Sprinkle chia seeds.

Cran-Apple Walnut Salad

Ingredients:

1-2 cups mixed greens

½ apple, sliced

¼ cup walnuts, chopped

¼ cup cranberries, dried or fresh

¼ cup yogurt

Instructions:

Mix together ingredients. Drizzle yogurt on top. Serve fresh.

Warm Brussel Sprouts Quinoa Salad

Ingredients:

1 cup brussels sprouts, sliced thinly

1 cup cooked quinoa

½ cup dried cranberries

¼ cup canned pumpkin

¼ cup chopped pecans

¼ cup black oil sunflower seeds

Instructions:

Mix together Brussel sprouts, quinoa, and cranberries. Drop dollop of canned pumpkin on top. Sprinkle pecans and sunflower seeds.

Rainbow Salad

Ingredients:

½ cup collard greens, chopped

¼ cup beets, chopped

¼ lima beans

1 tbsp black oil sunflower seeds

1 tbsp almond slices

Instructions:

Arrange all ingredients. Serve fresh.

Power Green Salad

Ingredients:

½ cup mustard greens, chopped

¼ cup green beans

¼ cup radishes, chopped

1 tsp chia seeds

Instructions:

Arrange all ingredients. Serve fresh.

Blueberry Dandelion Salad

Ingredients:

½ cup dandelion greens, chopped

¼ cup arugula

Handful of blueberries

3 cherry tomatoes

2 tsp chia seeds

Instructions:

Arrange all ingredients. Serve fresh.

Black Bean Salad

Ingredients

1 cucumber, diced

½ cup black beans, cooked

¼ cup corn, fresh or frozen

2 cherry tomatoes

Instructions:

Arrange all ingredients. Serve fresh.

Apple Cranberry Walnut Salad

Ingredients:

½ cup swiss chard

½ apple sliced

¼ cup yogurt

Pinch of walnuts

Pinch of cranberries, fresh or dried

Instructions:

Arrange all ingredients. Serve fresh.

Spinach Pumpkin Salad

Ingredients:

1 cup spinach

¼ cup canned pumpkin

¼ cup seed or nut mixture

Instructions:

Arrange all ingredients. Serve fresh.

Sunshine Salad

Ingredients:

½ cup bok choy, chopped

¼ cup radicchio, chopped

Orange slices

2 tbsp almond slices

Instructions:

Arrange all ingredients. Serve fresh.

Swiss Chard Salad

Ingredients:

½ cup swiss chard, chopped

¼ cup shredded carrots

2 tbsp walnuts

Instructions:

Arrange all ingredients. Serve fresh.

Sunday Salad

Ingredients:

¼ cup endive

¼ cup brussels sprouts

¼ cup radicchio, chopped

Instructions:

Arrange all ingredients. Serve fresh.

Monday Salad

Ingredients:

½ cup romaine lettuce, chopped

3 cherry tomatoes

Instructions:

Arrange all ingredients. Serve fresh.

Tuesday Salad

Ingredients:

½ cup power greens

1 diced tomato

Instructions:

Arrange all ingredients. Serve fresh.

Wednesday Salad

Ingredients:

½ cup leafy greens

Instructions:

Arrange all ingredients. Serve fresh.

Thursday Salad

Ingredients:

½ cup kale

¼ cup radish, chopped

Instructions:

Arrange all ingredients. Serve fresh.

Friday Salad

Ingredients:

½ cup collard greens

¼ cup radicchio, chopped

Instructions:

Arrange all ingredients. Serve fresh.

Saturday Salad

Ingredients:

½ cup bok choy

3 cherry tomatoes

1/4

Instructions:

Arrange all ingredients. Serve fresh.

CHAPTER 12

BREAKFAST

Barley Breakfast Bowl

Ingredients:

1 cup pearled barley

3 to 4 cups water

Instructions:

Combine barley and water in a sauce pan over the stove. Bring to a boil, then reduce heat and simmer for 25 minutes. Drain excess water. Serve topped with coconut oil, cranberries, and chia seeds.

Apple Barley Breakfast

Ingredients:

½ cup cooked barley

½ cup rolled oats

½ apple, diced

¼ cup pecans

Instructions:

Combine all ingredients. Serve fresh.

Quinoa Fruity Salad

Ingredients:

½ cup mixed fruit: mango, strawberry, blackberries, blueberries

½ cup leafy greens, chopped

¼ cup quinoa

Instructions:

Combine all ingredients, stir well. Serve fresh.

Quinoa Chia Porridge

Ingredients:

¾ cup quinoa, cooked with almond milk

3-5 almonds

1 tbsp coconut oil

2 tbsp chia seeds

Coconut flakes to top

Instructions:

Combine all ingredients. Serve fresh.

Quinoa Breakfast Bowl

Ingredients:

1 cup quinoa cooked with almond milk

¼ cup blueberries & raspberries

Instructions:

Top cooked quinoa with berries. Serve fresh.

Zucchini Breakfast Bowl

Ingredients:

½ cup shredded zucchini

½ banana, sliced

2 tbsp walnuts, chopped

1 tbsp chia seeds

Instructions:

Combine ingredients, serve fresh.

Pumpkin Coconut Oatmeal

Ingredients:

1 cup uncooked rolled oats

½ cup pureed pumpkin

½ cup water

2 tbsp coconut oil

Instructions:

Mix ingredients together. Microwave for 1 minute. Allow to cool, stir, and serve.

Strawberry Almond Oatmeal

Ingredients:

½ cup uncooked rolled oats

1 cup water

¼ cup sliced strawberries

Sliced almonds

Instructions:

Mix water and oats in bowl. Microwave for 45 seconds to 1 minute. Stir well. Top with strawberries and almond slices.

Scrambled Cauliflower

Ingredients:

1 cup cauliflower florets

1-2 eggs

1 tsp olive oil

Instructions:

Heat oil in skillet over high heat. Add cauliflower and stir to coat with oil. Sauté for 5 minutes. Add in eggs and stir until cooked thoroughly. Remove from heat, allow to cool, and serve fresh.

Mini Veggie Frittatas

Ingredients:

2 eggs

2 egg whites

¼ cup chopped spinach

¼ cup diced tomato

Instructions:

Preheat oven to 375 degrees. In a small mixing bowl, whisk together all ingredients. Pour mixture into muffin pan lined with muffin papers. Bake 20 minutes or until the centers of frittatas are firm. Freeze leftovers for another meal.

Pumpkin Quinoa Quiche

Ingredients:

1 cup cooked quinoa

1 cup milk

2 large eggs

1 cup canned pumpkin puree

1 cup spinach, chopped

Instructions:

Preheat oven to 350 degrees. Coat 8 inch baking pan with nonstick spray. Mix together all ingredients using a whisk. Pour mixture into pan. Bake for 45-50 minutes or until done. Remove from heat, allow to cool, separate into individual servings and freeze extras.

Peach and Black Bean Salsa

Ingredients:

1 peach, pitted and diced

¼ cup black beans, cooked

¼ cup beets, diced

2 tbsp fresh oregano leaves, chopped

Instructions:

Combine all ingredients. Serve fresh or top over a bed of mixed greens.

Make Ahead Pumpkin Oats

Ingredients:

½ cup rolled oats

½ cup almond milk

¼ cup toppings (pumpkin seeds, pecans, cranberries)

Instructions:

Place oats and milk in a mason jar with lid. Shake to combine ingredients well. Place in fridge overnight. In the morning, heat oats and sprinkle on toppings.

Red & Green Mini Pig Egg Cup

Ingredients:

5 eggs

¼ cup chopped spinach

¼ cup diced tomatoes

2 tbsp chia seeds

Instructions:

Preheat oven to 350 degrees. In small bowl, whisk eggs. Arrange additional ingredients in greased muffin pans. Pour egg mixture into each muffin pan. Bake for 20 minutes or until set. Allow to cool. Serve fresh & freeze extra portions for later meals.

Broccoli Carrots Mini Pig Egg Cup

Ingredients:

5 eggs

¼ cup diced broccoli

¼ cup shredded carrots

2 tbsp chia seeds

Instructions:

Preheat oven to 350 degrees. In small bowl, whisk eggs. Arrange additional ingredients in greased muffin pans. Pour egg mixture into each muffin pan. Bake for 20 minutes or until set. Allow to cool. Serve fresh & freeze extra portions for later meals.

Peas & Carrots Mini Pig Egg Cup

Ingredients:

5 eggs

¼ cup peas

½ cup carrots

¼ cup corn

Instructions:

Preheat oven to 350 degrees. In small bowl, whisk eggs. Arrange additional ingredients in greased muffin pans. Pour egg mixture into each muffin pan. Bake for 20 minutes or until set. Allow to cool. Serve fresh & freeze extra portions for later meals.

Pumpkin Spinach Mini Pig Egg Cup

Ingredients:

5 eggs

¼ cup canned pumpkin

¼ cup zucchini, diced

¼ cup spinach

Instructions:

Preheat oven to 350 degrees. In small bowl, whisk eggs. Arrange additional ingredients in greased muffin pans. Pour egg mixture into each muffin pan. Bake for 20 minutes or until set. Allow to cool. Serve fresh & freeze extra portions for later meals.

Baked Oatmeal Mini Pig Cups

Ingredients:

2 eggs

½ cup applesauce

1 ½ cup almond milk

3 cups rolled oats

Optional Toppings

Instructions:

Preheat oven to 350 degrees. Mix together ingredients. Pour into paper lined baking pan. Top with choice of toppings: seeds, nuts, or fruits. Press toppings firmly into oatmeal mixture. Bake 30 minutes. Allow to cool. Serve fresh or freeze for later meals.

Sunny Side Up Salad

Ingredients:

1 cup spinach

1 tomato, sliced

1 fried egg

Instructions:

Arrange ingredients on plate, serve fresh.

Eggs & Rice

Ingredients

½ cup leftover brown rice and/or barley

1 egg

1 tbsp coconut oil

Instructions: Heat oil in skillet. Add rice and/or barley. Stir until heated. Add egg, scramble until cooked. Serve fresh.

Banana Clove Pancakes

Ingredients

1 banana, ripe & mashed

½ cup rolled oats, blended to powder

1/3 cup almond milk

1 tsp baking powder

1 tsp cloves

Instructions:

Combine all ingredients. Pour over nonstick skillet cooking spray or coconut oil to prevent sticking. Cook until light brown, flip, pancakes, and continue cooking another 1-2 minutes. Serve fresh or freeze small portions for training treats.

CHAPTER 13

LUNCHES

Honey Roasted Parsnips & Carrots

Ingredients:

1 tbsp olive oil

2 tbsp honey

½ cup chopped parsnips

½ cup chopped carrots

Instructions:

Heat oven to 450 degrees. Toss to coat parsnips and carrots with oil and honey. Arrange vegetables on parchment paper lined baking sheet. Bake for 15-25 minutes or until vegetables are tender.

Roasted Cauliflower

½ cauliflower head, cut into small florets

2 tablespoons olive oil or melted coconut oil

Instructions:

Preheat oven to 425 degrees. Coat cauliflower with oil. Arrange on a baking sheet with parchment paper. Bake 15 minutes or until cauliflower is tender and tips are slightly brown. Allow to cool and serve.

Cranberry Infused Brussel Sprouts

Ingredients:

2 tbsp olive oil or melted coconut oil

1 cup brussels sprouts, cut in half

¼ cup cranberries, fresh or dried

Instructions:

Preheat oven to 400 degrees. Coat brussels sprouts and cranberries in oil. On parchment paper lined baking sheet, arrange brussels sprouts and cranberries. Bake for 15-25 minutes.

Zucchini and Corn Succotash

Ingredients:

1 tbsp coconut oil

1 zucchini, diced

¼ cup corn

¼ cup cooked black beans or lima beans

Instructions:

In skillet, heat oil. Add remaining ingredients. Sauté for 5-10 minutes or until food is warmed throughout. Remove from heat, allow to cool, serve fresh.

Coconut Roasted Baby Carrots

Ingredients:

1 cup baby carrots

1 tbsp coconut oil

½ tsp chia seeds

Instructions:

Preheat oven to 425 degrees. In mixing bowl, coat baby carrots with oil. Place carrots on parchment paper lined baking sheet. Bake for 15-20 minutes or until carrots are tender. Remove from oven and sprinkle chia seeds on carrots. Allow to cool, serve fresh.

Broccoli Stuffed Sweet Potato

Ingredients:

1 sweet potato, baked

½ cup broccoli florets, steamed

2 tbsp coconut oil

1 tbsp chia seeds

1 tbsp sliced almonds

Instructions:

Slice open sweet potato, stuff with broccoli. Drizzle melted coconut oil over broccoli and top with almonds and chia seeds.

Roasted Fall Vegetables

Ingredients:

½ cup cauliflower, cut into small florets

½ cup brussels sprouts, cut in half

½ cup baby carrots

2 tbsp coconut oil, melted

Instructions:

Preheat oven to 400 degrees. Coat vegetables with coconut oil. Place vegetables on parchment paper lined baking sheet. Bake for 15-25 minutes.

Zucchini Corn Black Bean Mix Up

Ingredients:

1 cup chopped zucchini

½ cup frozen corn, thawed

¼ cup black beans, or other beans, cooked

Instructions:

Combine all ingredients. Serve fresh.

Honey Glazed Carrots and Brussels Sprouts

Ingredients:

1 cup baby carrots, chopped

½ cup brussels sprouts, chopped

2 tbsp olive oil

2 tbsp honey

Instructions:

Warm oil in large skillet over medium heat. Add carrots, brussels sprouts, and honey. Cook, stirring occasionally, coating vegetables with oil and honey. Continue cooking for 10-15 minutes, or until desired tenderness. Serve fresh.

Eggplant Bulgar Lunch

½ cup bulgar wheat, cooked

½ eggplant, sliced thin

½ cup cherry tomatoes

Coconut oil

Instructions:

Brush eggplant slices with coconut oil. Arrange eggplant slices in single layer on baking sheet. Broil eggplant for 2 to 3 minutes. On plate, arrange bulgar, topped with eggplant slices and tomatoes.

Garbanzo Stir Fry

Ingredients:

1 cup garbanzo beans, cooked

½ zucchini, chopped

½ cup green beans

1 carrot, chopped

½ cup broccoli, chopped

2 tbsp coconut oil

½ cup cooked grain mixture: brown rice, barley, and bulgar

Instructions:

Heat oil in skillet over high heat. Stir in beans and vegetables. Cook until desired tenderness is reached. Serve over a bed of cooked grains.

Roasted Vegetables

Ingredients:

½ cup broccoli florets

1 cup butternut squash, chopped

½ zucchini, chopped

½ cup green beans

1 carrot, chopped

1 tomato, chopped

2 tbsp oil

Instructions:

Preheat oven to 425 degrees. Toss vegetables in oil to coat. Arrange on parchment paper lined baking sheet. Bake for 15 minutes. Allow to cool before serving. Refrigerate or freeze extra portions.

Green Beans with Cranberries

Ingredients:

1 cup green beans

¼ cup cranberries, fresh or dried

½ cup sliced almonds

Coconut oil

Instructions:

Preheat oven to 425 degrees. Mix all ingredients, coating with coconut oil. Arrange on parchment paper lined baking sheet. Bake for 15 minutes.

Ginger Lentils

Ingredients:

½ cup lentils, cooked

1 tbsp coconut oil

2 tbsp ginger root, freshly grated

1 tbsp sesame seeds

Instructions:

Combine lentils, coconut oil, and ginger in serving dish. Sprinkle sesame seeds over top. Serve fresh.

Nutty Butternut Squash

Ingredients

1 cup butternut squash, diced

½ cup apple cider or apple juice

¼ cup chopped pecans

2 tbsp ginger root, freshly grated

Instructions:

On stovetop deep sided skilled add all ingredients. Heat over medium high heat.

Bring to a boil, then reduce heat and simmer for 15-25 minutes or until tender, stirring gently. Remove from heat and serve fresh over a bed of brown rice and quinoa (optional).

Stir Fry Ginger Mustard Greens

Ingredients:

1 bunch mustard greens, chopped with stems

1 large tomato, diced

1 cup corn, fresh or frozen

2 tbsp ginger

¼ cup apple cider vinegar

2 tbsp olive oil

Instructions:

On stovetop, heat oil in deep sided skillet. Stir in greens, tomato, corn, ginger, and cider vinegar. Simmer over medium high heat, stirring occasionally. Add water by tablespoons if greens become too dry. Continue cooking greens down for about 10 minutes. Serve fresh or freeze into serving size portions.

Leafy Green Power Lunch

Ingredients:

2 cups swiss chard, chopped

2 cups spinach, chopped

1 tbsp coconut oil

2 tbsp water or apple cider vinegar

1-2 tbsp fresh herbs chopped (optional)

1 tbsp chia seeds

1 tbsp wheat germ

Instructions:

On stovetop, heat oil in deep sided skillet. Stir in greens. Simmer over medium high heat, stirring occasionally. Add water by tablespoons if greens become too dry. Continue cooking greens down for about 10 minutes. Remove from heat. Sprinkle chia seeds, herbs, and wheat germ over top. Serve fresh or freeze into serving size portions.

Spaghetti Squash

Ingredients:

1 spaghetti squash

Coconut oil

½ cup water

Instructions:

Cut spaghetti squash lengthwise. Scoop out seeds, feed to pig or save for another snack. Place spaghetti squash lengths, cut side down, into baking dish. Add water to dish. Bake at 375 for 30 minutes. Remove from oven. Rake fork along the inside of squash to pull apart the strands (spaghetti). Drizzle coconut oil over the top. Serve fresh or store extra portions in refrigerator.

Summer Fun Lunch

Ingredients:

¼ cup beans, cooked

½ yellow squash, sliced

½ cup zucchini, sliced

1 tomatoes, diced

1 tbsp coconut oil

½ cup brown rice, cooked

Instructions:

On stovetop, heat coconut oil over medium high heat. Stir in beans, squash, zucchini, and tomatoes. Cook until vegetables are tender. Serve over a bed of cooked brown rice.

Protein Power Lunch

Ingredients:

4 cups leafy greens (spinach, collard greens, mustard greens, etc)

¼ cup white beans, cooked

¼ cup lentils, cooked

¼ cup apple cider vinegar

2 tbsp almonds

Instructions:

On stovetop, simmer apple cider vinegar and leafy greens over high medium high heat. Stir occasionally. Once greens are cooked down, add in beans and lentils. Continue cooking an additional 5 minutes, or until heated through. Remove from heat, top with sliced almonds. Serve fresh or refrigerate additional portions.

CHAPTER 14

DINNER

AMPA Natural Diet Grain Mixture (COOKED)– Use For Multiple Recipes

Ingredients:

1 part brown rice

1 part lentils

1 part beans

1 part rolled oats

1 part barley

1 part wheat

Instructions:

Cook all foods per package directions. Once cooked and cooled, mix all ingredients together and store portion sizes in freezer for freshness. A large batch can be made and rationed out over time with the listed proportions. This has a higher protein content than the AMPA Natural Diet Dry Mixture (Enrichment) due to the lentils and beans. Serve appropriate portion as a meal or include in the following recipes.

AMPA Natural Diet Dry Mixture

Ingredients:

1 part wheat

1 part milo

1 part barley

1 part quinoa

1 part nuts & seeds: chia seeds, sesame seeds, almonds, pumpkin seeds, etc

1 part black oil sunflower seeds

2 parts rolled oats

Instructions:

Serve appropriate portion as a meal, incorporate into the following recipes, or use in enrichment activities for a meal on the go!

Slow Cooker Wheat Berries

Ingredients:

4 cups water

½ cup cooked lima beans

½ cup cooked black beans

½ cup dry wheat berries

1 cup diced tomatoes

Instructions:

Using a 3-4 quart slow cooker, add water and wheat berries. Cover and cook on high for 3 hours. Turn off heat. Stir in lima beans and black beans. Strain out excess water and serve fresh or freeze into individual portions.

Chickpea Tabbouleh

Ingredients:

½ cup bulgur wheat, cooked

½ cup chickpeas, cooked

4 tbsp fresh mint, minced

½ cucumber, diced

1 tomato, diced

Instructions:

Mix ingredients together, serve fresh.

Fiesta Burrito Bowl

Ingredients:

1 cup chopped leafy greens

½ cup AMPA Natural Diet Grain Mixture, cooked

½ tomato, diced

¼ cup corn, fresh or frozen

1 tbsp cilantro, chopped

Instructions:

Combine all ingredients in serving dish. Serve fresh.

Summer Grilled Burrito Bowl

Ingredients:

½ cup AMPA Natural Diet Grain Mixture, cooked

½ grilled zucchini, sliced

½ grilled yellow squash, sliced

¼ grilled eggplant, sliced

1 grilled radicchio

½ grilled tomato

1 tbsp cilantro, chopped

Instructions:

Combine all ingredients in serving dish. Serve fresh.

Lettuce Wrap Bowls

Ingredients:

Bibb or Boston lettuce leaves

½ cup AMPA Natural Diet Grain Mixture, cooked

¼ cup diced tomatoes

¼ cup shredded carrots

Almonds, sliced

Instructions:

On serving dish, arrange lettuce leaves. Add grain mixture to each. Top with tomatoes, carrots, and almonds. Serve fresh.

Eggplant Barley Dinner

Ingredients:

¼ to ½ eggplant, diced

1 cup spinach

½ cup barley, cooked

2 tbsp chia seeds

Instructions:

On serving dish, arrange spinach leaves. Top with barley, eggplant, and chia seeds. Serve fresh.

Spaghetti Squash Dinner Bowl

Ingredients:

1 spaghetti squash

½ cup water

1 cup purple cabbage, thinly sliced

¼ cup black beans, cooked

½ cup AMPA Natural Diet Grain Mixture, cooked

Instructions:

Cut spaghetti squash lengthwise. Scoop out seeds, feed to pig or save for another snack. Place spaghetti squash lengths, cut side down, into baking dish. Add water to dish. Bake at 375 for 30 minutes. Remove from oven. Rake fork along the inside of squash to pull apart the strands (spaghetti). Top squash with grain mixture, black beans, and cabbage. Serve fresh or freeze extra portions for later meals.

Texas Caviar

Ingredients:

1 cup black eyed peas, cooked

1 cup black beans, cooked

1 cup corn, fresh or frozen

1 cup tomato, chopped

½ cup purple cabbage, chopped

½ cup zucchini, chopped

Instructions:

Combine all ingredients. Serve fresh or refrigerate.

Pumpkin Puree Dinner

Ingredients:

1 cup spinach

1 cup canned pumpkin

1 cup cooked AMPA Natural Diet Grain Mixture

¼ cup walnuts

Instructions:

Spread spinach on serving dish. Spoon pumpkin onto spinach. Top with AMPA Natural Diet Grain Mixture. Sprinkle walnuts over top.

Pumpkin Black Bean Salad

Ingredients:

½ cup baby spinach leaves

1 cup fresh or frozen pumpkin chopped into cubes

½ cup cooked black beans

½ cup green beans, fresh or frozen

¼ cup cranberries, fresh or frozen

2 tbsp chia seeds

2 tbsp almonds

Instructions:

In serving dish, stir spinach, pumpkin cubes, black beans, and green beans together. Top with cranberries, chia seeds, and almonds.

Stuffed Acorn Squash

Ingredients:

1 cup brussels sprouts

1 acorn squash

1 cup cooked AMPA Natural Diet Grain Mixture

2 tbsp dry oats

2 tbsp cranberries, fresh or frozen

Instructions:

Preheat oven to 400 degrees. Slice acorn squash in half. Scoop out seeds if desired and save for a snack. Place in a baking dish with ½ inch water to prevent burning edges, cut side facing down. Brush olive oil or coconut oil on exposed areas of squash. Bake for one hour. Then allow to cool.

Slice brussels sprouts in halves and coat with oil. Arrange on a separate baking sheet. Roast at 400 degrees for 15 minutes. Allow to cool.

Using ½ squash as an edible bowl, mix in brussels sprouts and cooked AMPA Natural Diet Grain Mixture. Top with dry oats and cranberries.

Eggplant Chickpea Bake

Ingredients:

½ eggplant, sliced

½ cup chickpeas, cooked

½ cup AMPA Natural Diet Grain Mixture, cooked

2 tbsp coconut oil, melted

1 tomato, sliced

2 tbsp fresh basil, sliced

Instructions:

Preheat oven to 350 degrees. In baking dish, coat eggplant slices in melted coconut oil then arrange in single layer. Top with chickpeas, AMPA Natural Diet Grain Mixture, and sliced tomatoes. Bake for 15-20 minutes. Remove from oven and sprinkle with basil.

Egg Fried Rice & More

Ingredients:

1 cup AMPA Natural Diet Grain Mixture, cooked

½ cup baby carrots, sliced or chopped

½ cup peas, cooked

2 tbsp vegetable oil

1 egg

Instructions:

Heat oil skillet on medium-high heat. Pour in vegetables and egg, stirring briskly to scramble egg. Continue cooking until egg is well cooked. Mix in grains. Stir until thoroughly heated. Serve fresh.

Sprouted Lentils Dish

Ingredients:

½ cup sprouted lentils

2 tbsp sesame seeds

¼ cup chickpeas, cooked

½ cup AMPA Natural Diet Grain Mixture, cooked

½ small tomato, diced

¼ cup diced celery

½ cup leafy greens

Instructions:

On a bed of leafy greens, layer grain mixture, chickpeas, tomato, celery, sprouted lentils, and sesame seeds. Serve fresh.

Spinach Rice Balls

Ingredients:

1 cup frozen spinach leaves, thawed

1 cup cooked rice

1 large egg

2 tbsp olive oil

Instructions:

Preheat oven to 350 degrees. In medium skillet, heat oil over medium heat. Stir in spinach, cooking for 2 minutes. Combine egg, spinach, and rice in bowl. Form rounded tablespoon balls of mixture. Place balls on parchment paper lined baking sheet. Bake for 10 minutes. Allow to cool and serve fresh.

Stuffed Bell Peppers

Ingredients:

1-2 red or yellow bell peppers

1 carrot, diced

1 zucchini, diced

2 tbsp coconut oil

1 cup brown rice, cooked OR AMPA Natural Diet Grain Mixture, cooked

Instructions:

Preheat oven to 350 degrees. Slice tops off peppers. Use spoon to remove seeds, then replace tops. Place in oven safe dish and bake for 20 minutes. On stovetop, sauté carrots and zucchini in coconut oil for 6-7 minutes. Stir in cooked rice or grain mixture. Stuff mixture into pepper(s), overstuffing and then placing the top back on. Bake an additional 30 minutes. Allow to cool and serve.

Loaded Sweet Potatoes

Ingredients:

1 sweet potato, baked

¼ cup black beans, cooked

¼ cup black oil sunflower seed sprouts

2 tbsp chia seeds

¼ cup broccoli florets chopped

1 cup AMPA Natural Diet Grain Mixture, cooked

Instructions:

Slice baked sweet potato in half. Use fork to fluff up inside of potato. Top with black beans, sunflower sprouts, and then chia seeds.

On serving dish, next to sweet potato, stir together broccoli florets and grain mixture.

Broccoli Rice Gourmet

Ingredients:

¾ cup steamed broccoli, chopped

1 ½ cup AMPA Natural Diet Grain Mixture, cooked

2 tbsp coconut oil

2 tbsp sprouted black oil sunflower seeds

Instructions:

Heat coconut oil in skillet over medium heat. Sauté broccoli for 2 minutes, then stir in grain mixture. Stir occasionally for 5 minutes. Pour onto serving dish, top with sprouts.

Mushroom Rice Gourmet

Ingredients:

¾ cup button mushrooms, sliced

1 ½ cup AMPA Natural Diet Grain Mixture, cooked

2 tbsp coconut oil

2 tbsp sprouted lentils

Instructions:

Heat coconut oil in skillet over medium heat. Sauté mushrooms until soft, then stir in grain mixture. Stir occasionally for 5 minutes. Pour onto serving dish, top with sprouts.

Spinach Mushroom Dinner

Ingredients:

¾ cup button mushrooms, sliced

1 cup fresh or frozen spinach, chopped

1 ½ cup AMPA Natural Diet Grain Mixture, cooked

2 tbsp coconut oil

2 tbsp sesame seeds or flax seeds

Instructions:

Heat coconut oil in skillet over medium heat. Sauté mushrooms and spinach until soft, then stir in grain mixture. Stir occasionally for 5 minutes. Pour onto serving dish, top with seeds.

Artichoke Stuffed Eggplant

Ingredients:

1 eggplant, sliced lengthwise

6 ounces frozen artichoke hearts

1 cup spinach, chopped

1 cup AMPA Natural Diet Grain Mixture, cooked

2 tbsp hemp hearts

2 tbsp sliced almonds

1 tbsp olive oil

Instructions:

Preheat oven to 400 degrees. Scoop out middle of eggplant halves, leaving a border inside the skin to act as the bowl-shell. Drizzle olive oil inside eggplant halves. Place on parchment paper lined baking sheet. Coat scooped out eggplant and artichokes with olive oil and place on baking sheet next to eggplant halves. Bake until tender, then remove from oven. In large mixing bowl, combine scooped out eggplant, artichokes, spinach, and grain mixture. Scoop mixture into eggplant halves. Return baking sheet to oven. Bake stuffed eggplant for 10-15 minutes. Sprinkle hemp hearts and almonds to top.

Broccoli Cauliflower Bake

Ingredients:

2 cups broccoli, chopped

1 cup cauliflower, chopped

2 cups AMPA Natural Grain Mixture, cooked

½ cup chickpeas

½ cup chopped kale

¼ cup almond milk

¼ cup sliced almonds

Instructions:

In lightly greased glass baking dish, combine all ingredients except almonds. Sprinkle almonds on top then cover dish tightly with foil. Bake at 375 degrees for 30 minutes.

Quick Quinoa Dinner

Ingredients:

1 cup quinoa, cooked

1/2 cup leafy greens, chopped

1 tomato, diced

2 tbsp chia seeds

Instructions:

Mix all ingredients, serve.

Optional:

Serve alongside cooked or steamed green beans.

Mashed Cauliflower & Side Salad

Ingredients:

1 head of cauliflower

3 tbsp almond milk

Side salad with green beans

Instructions:

Chop cauliflower finely. Boil 2 cups water in sauce pan over high heat, add cauliflower, then reduce heat to medium. Cook for 15 minutes or until tender. Drain water thoroughly. In mixing bowl, combine milk and cauliflower. Mash with mashed potato masher. Serve with side salad with green beans.

Sweet Potato Casserole & Mixed Grains

Ingredients:

1 pound sweet potatoes, cooked

¼ cup almond milk

1 tsp cinnamon

1 tsp vanilla extract

¼ cup pecans, chopped

1 cup AMPA Natural Diet Grain Mixture, cooked

Instructions:

In large bowl, use mixer to whip sweet potatoes and milk. Pour mixture into glass baking dish. Sprinkle pecans over top. Bake covered at 350 degrees for 20 minutes.

Serve alongside grain mixture.

Bok Choy & Mixed Grains

Ingredients:

2 cups bok choy, chopped

1 cup AMPA Natural Diet Grain Mixture, cooked

2 tbsp flax seeds or hemp seeds

Instructions:

Stir together bok choy and grain mixture. Sprinkle seeds on top.

Roasted Asparagus & Sweet Potato with Grains

Ingredients:

1 cup asparagus, trimmed

1 cup sweet potatoes, chopped into small cubes

2 tbsp coconut oil

1 cup AMPA Natural Diet Grain Mixture, cooked

Instructions:

Coat asparagus and sweet potatoes in coconut oil. Bake in glass pan at 375 degrees for 20 minutes. Serve alongside grain mixture.

Sunflower Sprouts & Grains

Ingredients:

1 cup AMPA Natural Diet Grain Mixture, cooked

¼ cup black oil sunflower seed sprouts

Instructions:

Spread grain mixture on serving dish. Top with sprouts.

Brussel Sprouts & Radicchio

Ingredients:

½ cup brussel sprouts, chopped

½ cup radicchio, chopped

1 cup AMPA Natural Diet Grain Mixture, cooked

Instructions:

Combine all ingredients. Serve fresh.

White Bean & Sweet Potato Skillet

Ingredients:

1 tbsp olive oil

1 sweet potato, chopped into small cubes

½ cup white beans, cooked

1 tomato, chopped

1 cup baby spinach

1 cup AMPA Natural Diet Grain Mixture, cooked

Instructions:

Heat oil in skillet over high heat. Sauté sweet potatoes for 5-7 minutes. Stir in white beans, spinach, and tomatoes. Cook an additional 5 minutes or until heated through. Serve over a bed of grains.

Quinoa & Vegetables

Ingredients:

1 cup quinoa, cooked

1 tsp olive oil

½ cup black beans, cooked

½ cup zucchini, diced

½ cup yellow squash, diced

½ cup tomato, diced

½ cup corn kernels, frozen

1 cup kale

Instructions:

Heat oil in skillet over high heat. Sauté zucchini, squash, and corn for 5-7 minutes. Stir in black beans, tomatoes, and quinoa. Cook an additional 5 minutes or until heated through. Serve over a bed of kale.

Sweet Potato Chili

Ingredients:

2 sweet potatoes, cut into ½ inch cubes

1 tbsp olive oil

1 cup black beans, cooked

1 cup chickpeas, cooked

2 tomatoes, diced

2 tbsp ginger root, grated

1 tsp chili powder

½ cup water

2 cups AMPA Natural Diet Grain Mixture, cooked

¼ cup chia seeds

Instructions:

Coat nonstick skillet with cooking spray. Sauté sweet potato in olive oil for 5-7 minutes. Add in chili powder, ginger root,

black beans, chickpeas, tomatoes, and water. Bring to a boil, then reduce heat and simmer 30 minutes. Top with chia seeds. Serve over a bed of grain mixture.

Creamed Spinach and Parsnips

Ingredients:

2 tbsp coconut oil

1 tbsp vegetable oil

1 lb parsnips, cut into ½ to 1 inch pieces

½ cup low sodium vegetable broth

1 tsp thyme, chopped

10-ounce package frozen chopped spinach, thawed

1 tbsp flour

1 cup almond milk

½ tsp nutmeg

¼ cup sliced almonds

1 cup AMPA Natural Diet Grain Mixture, cooked

Instructions:

Heat 1 tsp coconut oil and vegetable oil over medium high heat in skillet. Add parsnips and cook for 8-10 minutes. Pour in vegetable broth. Bring to a boil, simmer for 10 minutes. Stir in thawed spinach.

In separate small saucepan, heat 1 tsp coconut oil, flour, almond milk, nutmeg, and thyme. Bring sauce to a boil, whisking for 2-4 minutes. Stir sauce into spinach and parsnips. Top with sliced almonds. Serve over a bed of mixed grains.

CHAPTER 15

DESSERTS

Strawberry Mousse

Ingredients:

½ cup melted coconut oil

1 large banana

6 strawberries

½ avocado (skinned and pit removed)

Instructions:

Place all ingredients in food processor or blender until smooth. To serve fresh, refrigerate 1 hour and enjoy. To save for individual servings, freeze in silicone molds or ice cube trays.

Fresh Breath Cinnamon Parfait Bites

Ingredients:

Yogurt, unsweetened

Mint leaves, chopped

Rolled oats

Cinnamon

Instructions:

In silicone molds or ice cube trays, pour a small amount of yogurt in each. Top with a pinch of each: mint leaves, rolled oats, and cinnamon. Refrigerate until solid. Store in fridge or freezer. Serve one treat daily.

Fresh Breath Parsley Mint Parfait Bites

Ingredients:

Yogurt, unsweetened

Mint leaves, chopped

Parsley, chopped

Rolled oats

Instructions:

In silicone molds or ice cube trays, pour a small amount of yogurt in each. Top with a pinch of each: mint leaves, rolled oats, and parsley. Refrigerate until solid. Store in fridge or freezer. Serve one treat daily.

Pumpkin Pie Bites

Ingredients:

½ cup canned pumpkin

½ cup melted coconut oil

Cinnamon

Clove

Nutmeg

Instructions:

In silicone molds or ice cube trays, press a small amount of canned pumpkin in each. Pour a layer of melted coconut oil over. Top with a pinch of cinnamon, clove, and nutmeg. Refrigerate until solid. Store in fridge or freezer. Serve one treat daily.

Pumpkin Walnut Parfait

Ingredients

¼ - ½ cup canned pumpkin

1 dollop yogurt

Cranberries, fresh or dried

Rolled oats, just a pinch

Instructions:

On serving dish, place pumpkin. Add dollop of yogurt. Top with cranberries and oats. Serve fresh.

Pineapple Raspberry Mint Parfait

Ingredients:

Yogurt

Raspberries, fresh or frozen

Pineapple, fresh or frozen, cubes

1 sprig mint leaves

Instructions:

In serving dish, layer ingredients. Serve fresh.

Berry Parfait

Ingredients:

½ cup yogurt

¼ cup berries, fresh or frozen

¼ cup rolled oats

Instructions:

In serving dish, pour yogurt. Top with berries and oats. Enjoy fresh!

Mango Blackberry Parfait

Ingredients:

Yogurt

Raspberries, fresh or frozen

Mango, fresh or frozen

1 sprig mint leaves

Sliced almonds

Rolled oats

Instructions:

In serving dish, layer ingredients. Serve fresh. Top with almonds and oats.

Apple Crisp

1 apple, cored and sliced thinly

Coconut oil

Cinnamon

Rolled oats

Instructions:

Sautee apple slices with coconut oil over high heat in skillet until softened. Serve with cinnamon and oats sprinkled on top.

Cinnamon Apples

Ingredients:

½ tbsp coconut oil

1 apple, sliced thinly

3 tbsp water

1 tbsp honey (optional)

1 tbsp chopped walnuts (optional)

Instructions:

Melt coconut oil in sauté pan over medium-high heat. Add apple slices, water, and honey. Stir gently and simmer for 8-12 minutes or until apple slices are tender. Remove from heat, allow to cool, and top with chopped walnuts before serving.

Fried Bananas

Ingredients:

1 Banana, sliced

1 tbsp coconut oil

Instructions:

Heat coconut oil in skillet over medium heat. Cook banana slices for 1-3 minutes on each side. Allow to cool, serve fresh.

Peach Cobbler

Ingredients:

1 can peaches, drained

½ cup rolled oats

1 dollop yogurt

Instructions:

On serving dish, arrange peaches, topped with rolled oats. Serve alongside a dollop of yogurt.

Grilled Pineapple

Ingredients:

Pineapple, sliced, fresh or canned & drained

Instructions:

Grill over medium heat for 2-3 minutes per side. Allow to cool. Serve fresh.

Grilled Ginger Peach Sundae

Ingredients:

Peaches, fresh, cut in half and pit removed

Pinch of ginger powder or freshly grated

Drizzle of honey

Instructions:

Place peaches, cut side down, on pre heated grill for 6 to 7 minutes or until golden brown. Place on serving dish. Drizzle sparingly with honey and a pinch of ginger.

Optional Whipped Coconut Oil Ice Cream:

In mixing bowl, beat ½ cup cold & solid unrefined coconut oil with 2 tbsp yogurt. Drop a dollop of ice cream into middle of grilled peach while warm. Allow to melt slightly.

Baked Pears

Ingredients:

1 pear, sliced in half lengthwise

½ cup rolled oats

¼ cup sliced almonds or chopped walnuts

1 tbsp coconut oil

Instructions:

Preheat oven t0 400 degrees. On baking sheet arrange pears, cut side up. Mix together oil, oats, and nuts. Bake 35-40 minutes. Allow to cool, serve fresh.

Honey Baked Nectarines

Ingredients:

Nectarine, cut in half with pig removed

1 tsp honey

½ tsp lemon juice

Instructions:

Preheat broiler. Place nectarines cut side up in baking pan. Combine honey and lemon juice, brush mixture over nectarines. Broil for 6-8 minutes. Serve warm with a dollop of yogurt.

Yogurt Tarts

Ingredients:

1 ¼ cup branflake or cornflake cereal

1 tbsp honey

¼ cup pecans, chopped

1 tbsp. coconut oil

¾ cup yogurt

½ cup fresh fruit

Instructions:

Preheat oven to 350 degrees. Place cereal flakes and pecans in food processor,

pulsing until well blended. Combine this mixture with honey and coconut oil. Press into 2 tart pans, forming bottom and sides of crust. Bake at 350 for 10 minutes. Remove from heat and allow to cool. Divide yogurt and fresh fruit between tarts.

Ginger Oranges

Ingredients:

Orange slices, fresh or canned & drained

Ginger root, grated

Instructions:

On serving dish, arrange orange slices. Sprinkle ginger root on top. Serve fresh.

No Bake Graham Cookies

Ingredients:

8 whole grain graham crackers, crushed and ground finely

¼ cup peanut butter

¼ cup chopped nuts

2 tbsp & 2 tsp honey

4 tsp shredded coconut

Instructions:

Combine all ingredients except shredded coconut, in a small bowl. Roll out small cookie balls and press lightly into shredded coconut to coat. Refrigerate until firm. Store in refrigerator for freshness.

Macadamia Cookie Dough

Ingredients:

½ cup coconut oil, melted

¼ cup macadamia nuts, chopped

Rolled oats

Cinnamon

Instructions:

In silicone molds or ice cube trays, pour a small amount of coconut oil in each. Top with a pinch of each: macadamia nuts, cinnamon, and rolled oats. Refrigerate until solid. Store in fridge or freezer. Serve one treat daily.

Yogurt Covered Strawberries

Ingredients:

Fresh strawberries with tops

½ cup coconut oil, melted

¼ cup yogurt

Instructions:

Combine coconut oil and yogurt. Dip bottoms of strawberries into mixture. Lay strawberries flat on parchment paper lined plate. Place in refrigerator until yogurt coating firms. Store in fridge, serve cold. TIP: Make sure coconut oil is hot to give you enough time to coat fruits. Chilled yogurt or pumpkin will cause the coconut oil to solidify and will be hard to spread onto fruit.

Optional Toppings:

After coating strawberries with yogurt mixture, sprinkle chia seeds, black oil sunflower seeds, or chopped nuts onto the soft mixture. Resume with instructions above, placing in refrigerator until firm.

Pumpkin Covered Bananas

Ingredients:

Banana, sliced thick

½ cup coconut oil

¼ cup canned pumpkin

Instructions:

Combine coconut oil and pumpkin. Dip bottoms of bananas into mixture, using toothpicks or forks as necessary for handling. Lay banana slices flat on parchment paper lined plate. Place in refrigerator until pumpkin coating firms. Store in fridge, serve cold. TIP: Make sure coconut oil is hot to give you enough time to coat fruits. Chilled yogurt or pumpkin will cause the coconut oil to solidify and will be hard to spread onto fruit.

Optional Toppings:

After coating banana slices with yogurt mixture, sprinkle chia seeds, black oil sunflower seeds, or chopped nuts onto the soft mixture. Resume with instructions above, placing in refrigerator until firm.

Yogurt Dipped Watermelon

Ingredients:

Watermelon triangle slices, with rind

½ cup coconut oil, melted

¼ cup yogurt

Instructions:

Combine coconut oil and yogurt. Dip tips of watermelon into mixture. Lay melon slices flat on parchment paper lined plate. Place in refrigerator until yogurt coating firms. Store in fridge, serve cold. TIP: Make sure coconut oil is hot to give you enough time to coat melon. Chilled yogurt or pumpkin will cause the coconut oil to solidify and will be hard to spread onto fruit.

Optional Toppings:

After coating watermelon slices with yogurt mixture, sprinkle chia seeds, black oil sunflower seeds, or chopped nuts onto the soft mixture. Resume with instructions above, placing in refrigerator until firm.

Frozen Watermelon Popsicles

Ingredients

Watermelon slices

Instructions:

Place watermelon slices on parchment paper lined baking sheet. If desired for human family members, poke popsicle stick into each watermelon slice. Place watermelon in freezer until frozen. Enjoy cold.

Melon Mint Smoothie

Ingredients:

2 cups watermelon pieces

½ cup ice

¼ cup coconut water

1 sprig mint

Instructions:

Blend all ingredients in blender. Serve fresh.

CHAPTER 16

BIRTHDAY BASH

Banana Birthday Cupcakes

Ingredients:

2 cups water

2 ripe bananas, mashed

3 cups flour

1 tbsp baking powder

1 egg

2 tbsp honey

1 tsp vanilla

1 tsp cinnamon

Instructions:

Preheat oven to 350 degrees. In bowl, combine all ingredients. Spoon into paper lined muffin pan. Bake for 20 minutes. Allow to cool.

Optional Frosting:

Blend together 4 ounces cream cheese at room temperature and 3 tbsp canned pumpkin.

Honey Peanut Butter Birthday Cupcakes

Ingredients:

2 eggs

1 ¾ cups flour

1 tsp baking powder

1 tsp baking soda

1 cup milk or almond milk

½ cup peanut butter

2 tbsp honey

¼ cup olive oil

Instructions:

Preheat oven to 350 degrees. In mixing bowl, combine all ingredients. Mix well. Spoon batter into paper lined cupcake pan. Bake 15-20 minutes. Allow cupcakes to cool.

Optional Frosting:

Mix together 1 mashed banana, 1 tbsp peanut butter, 3 tbsp carob powder, 1 tsp vanilla, 1 ½ tbsp flour, 1 tsp cinnamon. Spread onto cupcakes and top with a sprinkle of chopped pecans or rolled oats.

Apple Sweet Potato Birthday Cakes

Ingredients:

½ cup sweet potato, pureed

½ cup applesauce

1 tbsp honey

1 tbsp coconut oil

1 apple, grated

1 egg, beaten

¾ cups flour

2 tbsp rolled oats

Instructions:

Preheat oven to 350 degrees. In mixing bowl, combine all ingredients, wet ingredients first, then flour and rolled oats. Drop thickened dough into paper lined or greased mini muffin pans. Bake for 10-15 minutes. Allow to cool.

Optional Frosting:

Stir together 2 ounces softened cream cheese and 2 tbsp applesauce. Spread onto cupcakes. Top with sliced almonds.

Apple Cheddar Birthday Cupcakes

Ingredients:

2 eggs

½ cup unsweetened apple sauce

¼ cup vegetable oil

2 tbsp honey

1 cup apple, grated

½ cup cheese, shredded

1 ½ cups flour

½ cup rolled oats

2 tsp baking powder

½ tsp baking soda

Instructions:

Preheat oven to 350 degrees. In small bowl, combine wet ingredients. In separate large mixing bowl, combine dry ingredients. Stir wet ingredients into large bowl with dry ingredients. Pour batter into paper lined cupcake pan. Bake 15-20 minutes or until toothpick comes out clean.

Optional Frosting:

Stir together 2 ounces softened cream cheese and 2 tbsp applesauce. Spread onto cupcakes. Top with sliced almonds.

Carrot Cake Birthday Cupcakes

Ingredients:

2 cups carrots, shredded

3 eggs

½ cup applesauce

½ cup rolled oats

3 cups whole wheat flour

Instructions:

Preheat oven to 350 degrees. In mixing bowl, combine carrots, eggs, and applesauce. Stir in rolled oats and flour. Mix well. Pour thick mixture into paper lined muffin tins. Bake 25 minutes.

Optional Frosting:

Stir together 2 ounces softened cream cheese and 2 tbsp applesauce. Spread onto cupcakes. Top with shredded carrots.

Birthday Ice Cream Cake

Ingredients:

½ cup peanut butter

½ cup yogurt

1 banana, mashed

¼ cup melted coconut oil

Splash coconut water to desired consistency

Instructions:

Combine all ingredients. Pour ice cream into silicone muffin cups of various sizes. Freeze until solid. Remove ice cream cake layers from muffin cups. Stack ice cream layers and serve cold.

Mini Carrot Cakes

Ingredients:

½ cup flour

½ tsp baking powder

1 tbsp peanut butter

2 tbsp apple sauce

1 tsp vanilla

1 tbsp honey

1 egg

1 tbsp coconut oil, melted

¼ shredded carrots

Instructions:

Preheat oven to 350 degrees. Combine all ingredients in mixing bowl. Fill paper lined muffin cups with batter. Bake 15-20 minutes. Allow to cool.

Optional Frosting:

Beat 4 ounces softened cream cheese and ¼ cup canned pumpkin. Top with shredded carrots or rolled oats.

Apple Pumpkin Mini Muffins

Ingredients:

1 cup canned pumpkin

½ cup almond milk

3 cups rolled oats

1 apple, diced

Instructions:

Preheat oven to 350 degrees. In mixing bowl, combine all ingredients. Fill mixture into mini muffin pan sprayed with cooking spray. Press lightly to pack mixture into each muffin. Bake 15-25 minutes or until muffins pull away from sides of pan. Allow to cool, serve fresh or freeze extra portions to store.

Zucchini Birthday Mini Cakes

Ingredients:

½ cup shredded zucchini

1 egg

1 tsp olive oil or coconut oil

½ cup water

2 tbsp chia seeds

½ cup tapioca flour

¾ cup garbanzo bean flour

Instructions:

Preheat oven to 350 degrees. In mixing bowl, combine zucchini, egg, oil, chia seeds and water. Stir in flour until mixed well. Pour batter into silicone mini muffin baking molds filling each ½ way. Bake 20 minutes or until done. Allow to cool before removing from silicone molds.

Coconut Covered Fruit Birthday Bouquet

Ingredients:

Fresh strawberries with tops

Honey dew slices or balls

Cantaloupe slices or balls

Pineapple slices or cut shapes

Banana Slices

Grapes

½ cup coconut oil, melted

¼ cup yogurt and/or canned pumpkin

Instructions:

Combine coconut oil and yogurt or coconut oil and pumpkin. Use wooden kebab sticks to hold fruit. Dip various fruit pieces into coconut oil mixture. Poke sticks into floral foam inside mug, cup, or other container. Place in refrigerator until coconut oil coating firms. Store in fridge, serve cold, removing sticks before feeding fruits. TIP: Make sure coconut oil is hot to give you enough time to coat fruits. Chilled yogurt or pumpkin will cause the coconut oil to solidify and will be hard to spread onto fruit.

Optional Toppings:

After coating fruits with coconut oil mixture, sprinkle chia seeds, black oil sunflower seeds, or chopped nuts onto the soft

mixture. Resume with instructions above, placing in refrigerator until firm.

Pecan Pie Muffins

Ingredients:

½ cup light brown sugar

¼ cup flour

1 cup pecans, chopped

1/3 cup butter, softened

1 egg

Instructions:

Preheat oven to 350 degrees. In small mixing bowl, combine egg and butter. Stir well. Fold in brown sugar, flour, and pecans. Pour batter into 6 greased muffin tins. Bake 10-13 minutes.

Fruit Layer Birthday Cake

Ingredients:

Watermelon

Pineapple

Blueberries

Orange slices

Kiwi slice

Instructions:

Slice watermelon and and pineapple to different diameters and thickness for alternating layers. Stack layers. Arrange orange slices around bottom of cake. Arrange blueberries and kiwi slices where appropriate. Serve fresh.

Birthday Waffle Fruit Cups

Store bought waffle ice cream "cups"

Variety of chopped fruits and berries

Instructions:

Arrange fruit in waffle cups. Serve to each party guest, human or pig!

Kiwi Birthday Bites

Ingredients:

Kiwi, skinned and sliced

Yogurt

Raspberries

Instructions:

Arrange sliced kiwi on serving platter. Drop one dollop of yogurt in center of each. Top each kiwi with one raspberry. Serve fresh.

Watermelon Pizza

Ingredients:

Watermelon

Yogurt

Choice of fruit toppings

Chopped mint leaves

Shredded coconut

Instructions:

Slice 2-inch section of watermelon out of the middle to start a pizza base. Spread yogurt across, avoiding the edges for ease of grabbing slices. Top with choice of fruit toppings. Strawberries, blackberries, blueberries, kiwi, and pineapple are popular choices. Sprinkle chopped mint leaves and shredded coconut to garnish.

Pumpkin Pie Ice Cream

Ingredients:

1 cup yogurt

1 ripe banana

½ cup pumpkin puree

¼ cup coconut milk or coconut water

Instructions:

Combine ingredients in blender. Pour into individual serving size disposable cups. Place in freezer until frozen solid. Remove paper cup before serving. Enjoy!

Peanut Butter Banana Ice Cream

Ingredients:

1 cup yogurt

1 ripe banana

½ cup peanut butter

¼ cup coconut milk or coconut water

Instructions:

Combine ingredients in blender. Pour into individual serving size disposable cups. Place in freezer until frozen solid. Remove paper cup before serving. Enjoy!

Watermelon Ice Cream

Ingredients:

1 cup watermelon chunks

½ cup yogurt

¼ cup coconut milk or coconut water

Instructions:

Combine ingredients in blender. Pour into individual serving size disposable cups. Place in freezer until frozen solid. Remove paper cup before serving. Enjoy!

Strawberries & Cream Ice Cream

Ingredients:

1 cup strawberries

½ cup yogurt

¼ cup coconut milk or coconut water

Instructions:

Combine ingredients in blender. Pour into individual serving size disposable cups. Place in freezer until frozen solid. Remove paper cup before serving. Enjoy!

Coconut Ice Cream

Ingredients:

2 egg yolks

¼ cup apple sauce

1 – 13.5 oz can coconut milk

½ cup shredded coconut

Instructions:

In mixing bowl, whisk together applesauce and egg yolks. Add coconut milk, continue whisking. Over medium heat, pour mixture into pot. Cook for 10 minutes, stirring constantly while mixture thickens. Pour into clean mixing bowl. Freeze 30 minutes, then remove from freezer, beat mixture. Return to freezer for another 30 minutes, then beat again. Continue to freeze and beat mixture 2 more times for idea consistency.

Alternatively, after cooking on stovetop, pour into individual serving size disposable cups. Place in freezer until frozen solid. Remove paper cup before serving. Enjoy!

CHAPTER 17

ENRICHMENT

AMPA Natural Diet Dry Mixture

Ingredients:

1 part wheat

1 part milo

1 part barley

1 part quinoa

1 part nuts & seeds: chia seeds, sesame seeds, almonds, pumpkin seeds, etc

1 part black oil sunflower seeds

2 parts rolled oats

AMPA Mini Pig Trail Mix

Ingredients:

1 cup raw whole almonds

1 cup raw pumpkin seeds

1 cup black oil sunflower seeds

1 cup mix nuts, unsalted (almonds, peanut, walnuts, brazil nuts, cashews, hazelnuts, macadamia nuts, pine nuts,

1 cup banana chips

Instructions:

Store in airtight container and use as appropriate.

Mini Pig Seed Mix

Ingredients:

1 cup black oil sunflower seeds

1 cup raw pumpkin seeds

1 cup sesame seeds

1 cup chia seeds

1 cup quinoa

Instructions:

Store in airtight container and use as appropriate.

Store Bought Treat Dispensing Toys

Purchase treat dispensing toys on Amazon.com or any pet store. These toys are designed to roll, wobble, or create a puzzle to provide physical and mental enrichment for your while, dropping treats sparingly. Remember, the bigger the holes the more versatile it will be with different foods but the faster the food will come out! Less holes will be more challenging giving the pig more exercise and stimulation. A variety of toys with holes of different sizes for different treats and difficulty levels will keep your pig more entertained. Appropriate treats vary depending on type of toy and size of holes, but may include:

AMPA Natural Diet Dry Mixture, or any single ingredient

Mini Pig Trail Mix, or any single ingredient

Mini Pig Seed Mix, or any single ingredient

Rolled oats

Black oil sunflower seeds

Puffed rice cereal

Cheerios

3 or 5 Gallon Water Jug

Upcycle a 3 or 5-gallon hard plastic water jug that no longer holds water, or buy a new one for relatively low cost. Drill size appropriate holes around the sides and/or bottom of the jug. Remember, the bigger the holes the more versatile it will be with different foods but the faster the food will come out! Less holes will be more challenging giving the pig more exercise and stimulation. A variety of toys with holes of different sizes for different treats and difficulty levels will keep your pig more entertained.

Appropriate treats vary depending on size of holes, but may include:

AMPA Natural Diet Dry Mixture, or any single ingredient

Mini Pig Trail Mix, or any single ingredient

Mini Pig Seed Mix, or any single ingredient

Rolled oats

Black oil sunflower seeds

Webbed Rubber Ball

Webbed rubber balls such as the Hol-ee Roller may be purchased from Amazon.com or your local pet store. The open design of these toys allows you to stuff treats or healthy vegetables inside for a challenging meal. The pigs must work to get the food out. You can also stuff newspaper or cloth inside, crumpled up with grains, seeds, or treats.

Appropriate treats will vary depending on toy and purpose. Try stuffing with these:

Lettuce

Bok choy

Broccoli florets

Carrot sticks

Grass clippings

Whiffle Ball Toy

Using a plastic whiffle ball, tape over the majority of holes. Fill with treats. The pigs will roll the ball around, slowly dispensing the snacks.

Suspended Treat: Fresh Foods

Use one of the following foods for your Suspended Treat:

Banana

Pumpkin

Apple

Cucumber

Butternut Squash

Acorn Squash

Spaghetti Squash

Carrot

Parsnip

Beet

Kohlrabi

Using the food whole, or a large chunk of the food, string a piece of rope or twine through. Secure the other end of rope to a nearby tree, fence, or other structure, ensuring the food is at eye level for your pig. The suspended treat will provide your pig with mental and physical enrichment. As the food rolls away at each chomp, the pig will need to think on the best way to get the reward they are after!

The Great Pumpkin Challenge

Offer your pig a whole pumpkin. For the most challenge and enrichment, do not cut into the pumpkin or smash it. Allow the pig to roll it around, work at it, think about it, and find a way to get in. If your pig is not interested in the whole pumpkin or it proves too difficult you may cut a starter hole or smash it on the ground to put a crack in it. The entire pumpkin is edible, including the skin, the guts, the seeds, and the flesh. However, eating an excessive amount may cause digestive upset. For smaller pigs, a small pie pumpkin is appropriate for their first pumpkin challenge. Alternately, you may remove the pumpkin once they have

eaten a good portion. Refrigerate or freeze and offer it again the following day.

Frozen Swing Treats: Summer Delights

Ingredients:

Cranberry Juice

Cucumbers, diced

Blueberries

Mangos, diced

Additional Items:

Water

Twine, string, or rope, cut into lengths for hanging treats

Small food containers or bowls

Instructions:

Using portions of your choice, spread cucumbers, blueberries, and mangos in each container. Add a splash of cranberry juice to each. Then fill with water. Lastly, submerge part of twine, string, or rope in the water. This will secure your rope to the frozen treat, with the remaining section of rope serving as means to hang the treat. Carefully place food containers in freezer, taking care not to spill. Keep in freezer until frozen solid. Hang from tree, fence, or other outdoor place for an afternoon enrichment. The pig will enjoy chasing the frozen treat, nibbling at it, and licking the melting juice. As the sun melts the ice, the fruits and/or vegetables will drop down for pig to enjoy!

Frozen Swing Treats: Fall Feast

Ingredients:

Cranberry Juice

Cranberries

Pumpkin chunks

Additional Items:

Water

Twine, string, or rope, cut into lengths for hanging treats

Small food containers or bowls

Instructions:

Using portions of your choice, spread cranberries and pumpkin chunks in each container. Add a splash of cranberry juice to each. Then fill with water. Lastly, submerge part of twine, string, or rope in the water. This will secure your rope to the frozen treat, with the remaining section of rope serving as means to hang the treat. Carefully place food containers in freezer, taking care not to spill. Keep in freezer until frozen solid. Hang from tree, fence, or other outdoor place for an afternoon enrichment. The pig will enjoy chasing the frozen treat, nibbling at it, and licking the melting juice. As the sun melts the ice, the fruits and/or vegetables will drop down for pig to enjoy!

Frozen Swing Treats: Hydration Station

Ingredients:

Coconut water

Cucumbers, diced

Watermelon chunks

Additional Items:

Water

Twine, string, or rope, cut into lengths for hanging treats

Small food containers or bowls

Instructions:

Using portions of your choice, spread cucumber and watermelon pieces in each container. Add a splash of coconut water to each. Then fill with water. Lastly, submerge part of twine, string, or rope in the water. This will secure your rope to the frozen treat, with the remaining section of rope serving as means to hang the treat. Carefully place food containers in freezer, taking care not to spill. Keep in freezer until frozen solid. Hang from tree, fence, or other outdoor place for an afternoon enrichment. The pig will enjoy chasing the frozen treat, nibbling at it, and licking the melting juice. As the sun melts the ice, the fruits and/or vegetables will drop down for pig to enjoy!

Frozen Swing Treats: Cran-Apple Delight

Ingredients:

Coconut water

Cranberries

Apple, diced

Blueberries

Additional Items:

Water

Twine, string, or rope, cut into lengths for hanging treats

Small food containers or bowls

Instructions:

Using portions of your choice, spread cranberries, blueberries, and apple pieces in each container. Add a splash of coconut water to each. Then fill with water. Lastly, submerge part of twine, string, or rope in the water. This will secure your rope to the frozen treat, with the remaining section of rope serving as means to hang the treat. Carefully place food containers in freezer, taking care not to spill. Keep in freezer until frozen solid. Hang from tree, fence, or other outdoor place for an afternoon enrichment. The pig will enjoy chasing the frozen treat, nibbling at it, and licking the melting juice. As the sun melts the ice, the fruits and/or vegetables will drop down for pig to enjoy!

Frozen Swing Treats: Vitamin Power

Ingredients:

Coconut water

Orange slices

Blueberries

Mint leaves

Additional Items:

Water

Twine, string, or rope, cut into lengths for hanging treats

Small food containers or bowls

Instructions:

Using portions of your choice, spread blueberries, orange slices, and mint leaves in each container. Add a splash of coconut water to each. Then fill with water. Lastly, submerge part of twine, string, or rope in the water. This will secure your rope to the frozen treat, with the remaining section of rope serving as means to hang the treat.

Carefully place food containers in freezer, taking care not to spill. Keep in freezer until frozen solid. Hang from tree, fence, or other outdoor place for an afternoon enrichment. The pig will enjoy chasing the frozen treat, nibbling at it, and licking the melting juice. As the sun melts the ice, the fruits and/or vegetables will drop down for pig to enjoy!

Natural Foraging

Ingredients:

Your choice of AMPA Natural Diet Dry Mixture, AMPA Mini Pig Trail Mix, or your choice of vegetables, grains, nuts, seeds, or fresh air popped popcorn with no salt or butter. May include an egg on occasion; raw or boiled.

Instructions:

Sprinkle or hide foods around the yard and/or in the grass. For weight loss, use low calorie treats such as vegetables and spread out the food to encourage walking and exercise. Teach the pig to search for the food by placing small piles of food in the same places each time. As they learn to search for the food, scatter or place the food further apart.

Hide and Seek

Ingredients:

Your choice of AMPA Natural Diet Dry Mixture, AMPA Mini Pig Trail Mix, or your choice of vegetables, grains, nuts, seeds, or fresh air popped popcorn with no salt or butter.

Instructions:

Hide small piles of treats under objects giving the pigs an exciting game of hide and seek and the opportunity to use their snout to move items. Examples: under an upside-down plastic flowerpot, under or inside a shoe, under a doormat, under or on a chair seat, under an upside-down bucket, under or on top of kid's toys, under a step, or under a rock. Get creative!

For weight loss, use low calorie treats such as vegetables and spread out the food to encourage walking and exercise.

Rooting Box

Ingredients:

Your choice of AMPA Natural Diet Dry Mixture, AMPA Mini Pig Trail Mix, or your choice of grains, nuts, seeds, or fresh air popped popcorn with no salt or butter.

Instructions:

Sprinkle foods in a box filled with plastic ball pit balls, large river rocks, or pig-safe toys. The idea is to give the pigs a challenge, using their snout to move objects around to find their treats.

Hay Rooting

Ingredients:

Your choice of AMPA Natural Diet Dry Mixture, AMPA Mini Pig Trail Mix, or your choice of grains, nuts, seeds, or fresh air popped popcorn with no salt or butter.

Instructions:

Sprinkle or hide foods in a pile of hay. The hay pile can be simply piled up on the ground, can go into a rooting box, or in the bottom half of a large plastic airline crate.

Shuffle up the hay to allow the foods to fall into various areas giving the pigs more of a challenge.

PVC Tube Dispenser

Ingredients:

Your choice of AMPA Natural Diet Dry Mixture, AMPA Mini Pig Trail Mix, or your choice of grains, nuts, seeds, or fresh air popped popcorn with no salt or butter.

Instructions:

Cut a section of PVC pipe with cap ends. Drill holes throughout the pipe. Treats can be added inside the pipe. Then, the pig can roll the pipe around the yard OR it can be mounted to a frame to keep it in place, either indoors or outdoors. As the pig roots at the pvc pipe, it will rotate allowing the treats to drop through the holes. Start with minimum holes and increase holes as necessary to accommodate the challenge level your pig desires.

Kiddy Pool

Ingredients:

Any food or snacks. Floating foods are easier to entice pigs into the water. As they become more comfortable they may be willing to go under to get foods at the bottom. Lettuce and air popped popcorn are great

Instructions:

Pools are GREAT! Inflatable pools or hard plastic pools work unless your pig is a destructor. Many vegetables will float in the water. This is a great way to introduce your pig to the pool and make it rewarding. A pig can enjoy their pool in many ways: cooling off, splashing, flopping, hydrating, or munching on a floating salad. If your pig is particularly fond of the water you can even SINK treats and she will snorkel around the bottom of the pool!! If you have a hard plastic pool and your pig hesitates to enter, try using a rubber bathmat with suction cups. It'll give then better traction and make them more comfortable.

CHAPTER 18

TRAINING TREATS

AMPA Ultimate Training Mix

Ingredients:

1/4 cup unsalted mixed nuts

1/4 cup unsalted almonds (optional)

1/4 cup black oil sunflower seeds

1/4 cup unsalted pumpkin seeds

1/4 cup dried coconut chunks

1/4 cup dried strawberry slices

Mix ingredients and store in airtight container. Perfect for training treats, on the go rewards, recall training, and harness training.

Apple Chip Training Treats:

Ingredients:

1 medium apple, cored and sliced extra thin

Instructions:

Preheat oven to 200 degrees. Arrange apple slices in a single layer on parchment lined baking sheet. Bake for one hour. Flip apples. Bake 1-2 more hours, flipping every 15 minutes, until apples are dry and crispy. Remove from heat. Cool completely and then store in airtight container. May also be stored in freezer.

Power Snack Training Mix

Ingredients:

1 cup cheerios

¾ cup almonds

¼ cup dried cranberries

¼ cup raw unsalted pumpkin seeds

¼ cup black oil sunflower seeds

Instructions:

Mix all ingredients together. Use for training treats.

Pumpkin Granola Bars

Ingredients:

1 tablespoons ground flaxseeds mixed with 2 tablespoons of warm water

½ cup pumpkin puree

1 cup rolled oats

½ cupped chopped nuts

½ cup dried fruit

Instructions:

Preheat oven to 350 degrees. Line a small baking pan or bread pan with parchment paper. Mix all ingredients and stir well. Spoon mixture into pan, pressing it flat and scoring into serving sizes. Bake 15-25 minutes or until edges begin to brown. Cut into serving portions. Allow to cool, enjoy fresh, freeze or refrigerate extra portions to preserve freshness.

Toasted Pumpkin Seeds

Ingredients:

1 cup fresh pumpkin seeds, rinsed

1 tbsp coconut oil, melted

Instructions:

Preheat oven to 350 degrees. Coat pumpkin seeds with coconut oil. Spread in single layer on parchment paper lined baking sheet. Bake 10-15 minutes, tossing occasionally.

Trail Mix No Bake Bites

Ingredients:

¼ cup chopped cranberries, fresh or dried

¼ cup walnuts, chopped

¼ cup sunflower seeds

½ cup rolled oats

2 tbsp chia seeds

¾ cup unsweetened coconut flakes

¼ ground flaxseed or brewers yeast

¾ cup natural creamy almond butter, unsalted

Instructions:

In large bowl, mix together all ingredients stirring well, then adding almond butter in last. Mix until uniform consistency. If too dry, add in a little more almond butter. Spoon out 1 tsp to 1 tbsp at a time, rolling into balls. Serve fresh, refrigerating or freezing remaining portions to preserve freshness.

Coconut Peanut Butter No Bake Bites

Ingredients:

½ cup shredded coconut

½ cup rolled oats

2 tbsp cup ground flaxseed

2 tbsp chia seeds

2 tbsp chopped macadamia or other nuts

½ cup natural peanut butter

2 tbsp honey

Instructions:

In large bowl, mix together all ingredients stirring well, then adding almond butter in last. Mix until uniform consistency. If too dry, add in a little more peanut butter. Spoon out 1 tsp to 1 tbsp at a time, rolling into balls. Serve fresh, refrigerating or freezing remaining portions to preserve freshness.

Coconut Cranberry No Bake Bites

Ingredients:

½ cup chopped cranberries, fresh or dried

¼ cup walnuts, chopped

½ cup rolled oats

2 tbsp chia seeds

1 cup unsweetened coconut flakes

¼ ground flaxseed or brewers yeast

¾ cup natural creamy almond butter, unsalted

¼ cup honey

Instructions:

In large bowl, mix together all ingredients stirring well, then adding almond butter in last. Mix until uniform consistency. If too dry, add in a little more almond butter. Spoon out 1 tsp to 1 tbsp at a time, rolling into balls. Serve fresh, refrigerating or freezing remaining portions to preserve freshness.

Oatmeal Raisin No Bake Bites

Ingredients:

½ cup raisins

¼ cup walnuts, chopped

¾ cup rolled oats

½ cup unsweetened coconut flakes

¼ ground flaxseed or brewers yeast

¾ cup natural creamy almond butter, unsalted

Instructions:

In large bowl, mix together all ingredients stirring well, then adding almond butter in last. Mix until uniform consistency. If too dry, add in a little more almond butter. Spoon out 1 tsp to 1 tbsp at a time, rolling into

balls. Serve fresh, refrigerating or freezing remaining portions to preserve freshness.

Cranberry Pumpkin Oat Cookies

Ingredients:

1 ¼ cup oats

½ cup pumpkin puree

½ cup dried cranberries, chopped

Instructions:

Preheat oven to 350 degrees. Mix all ingredients in bowl, stirring well. On parchment paper lined cookie sheet arrange tablespoon sized balls of dough, gently pressing a fork to flatten them into cookie shapes. Bake 10 minutes, allow to cool. Serve fresh or freeze to store in freezer.

Trail Mix Cookies

Ingredients:

¼ cup unrefined coconut oil, melted

2 tablespoons honey

2 eggs, beaten

½ cup canned pumpkin

1 cup rolled oats

1 cup quick cooking oats

½ cup cranberries, dried

½ cup raw pumpkin seeds

1 tsp pumpkin pit spice

¼ cup almonds, chopped

¼ cup ground flax seed

Instructions:

Preheat oven to 350 degrees. In small bowl, combine coconut oil, honey, eggs, spice and pumpkin. In separate bowl mix together oats, cranberries, pumpkin seeds, almonds, and flax seed. Stir dry ingredients together thoroughly, then fold in wet ingredients. Place tablespoon sized balls of dough onto parchment paper lined baking sheet. Flatten into desired shape, squares, circles, or use small cookie cutter to shape the dough. Bake for 15-20 minutes. Allow to cool, serve fresh, or freeze to preserve extras.

Apple Pecan Sunrise Cookies

Ingredients:

1 egg, beaten

¼ cup unsweetened apple sauce

2 tablespoons cup coconut oil, melted

½ cup diced apple

½ cup pecans, chopped

½ cup old fashioned oats

½ cup quick oats

Instructions:

Preheat oven to 350 degrees. In small bowl, stir together egg, apple sauce, and coconut oil. In separate bowl stir together oats, pecans, and apple pieces. Combine wet and dry ingredients, stirring thoroughly. Place tablespoon sized balls of dough onto parchment paper lined baking sheet. Flatten into desired shape, squares, circles, or use small cookie cutter to shape the dough. Bake for 15-20 minutes. Allow to cool, serve fresh, or freeze to preserve extras.

Peanut Butter Banana Breakfast Cookies

Ingredients:

¾ cup peanut butter

1 banana, mashed

¼ cup coconut oil, melted

¼ cup honey

¾ cup dried cranberries or other dried fruit

½ cup sunflower seeds

1 cup old fashioned oats

1 cup quick cooking oats

Instructions:

Preheat oven to 325 degrees. In mixing bowl, combine peanut butter, banana, coconut oil, and honey. Stir well. Fold in oats, cranberries, and sunflower seeds. Place tablespoon sized balls of dough onto parchment paper lined baking sheet. Flatten into desired shape, squares, circles, or use small cookie cutter to shape the dough. Bake for 15-20 minutes. Allow to cool, serve fresh, or freeze to preserve extras.

Pumpkin Bites

Ingredients:

1 ½ oat flour

2/3 cup canned pumpkin

1 egg

Instructions:

Preheat oven to 350 degrees. Combine ingredients in mixing bowl to form a stuff dough. If dough is too sticky, add flour. If dough is too dry, add water or pumpkin sparingly until workable. Lightly flour work area, roll dough to ¼ inch thick, and cut out small shapes with cookie cutters. On parchment paper lined baking sheet, bake cookies for 35 minutes or until crisp. Allow to cool, serve fresh or store in freezer for prolonged storage.

Banana Oat Training Cookies

Ingredients:

1 ½ cup flour

1 tsp baking powder

½ tsp baking soda

½ tsp cinnamon

1 ripe banana

1 egg

2 tsp olive oil

¼ cup applesauce

1 ¾ cup rolled oats

¾ cup dried cranberries

¾ cup pecans, chopped

Instructions:

Preheat oven to 350 degrees. In large bowl, mix together flour, baking powder, baking soda, and cinnamon. In separate bowl, mash banana. Stir in egg, oil, and applesauce. Slowly stir banana mixture into dry mixture. Fold in oats, pecans, and cranberries. Drop small balls of dough onto parchment paper lined baking sheet, 2 inches apart. Bake 12 to 15 minutes. Allow to cool. Serve fresh or store in freezer to preserve.

Pumpkin Peanut Butter Training Bites

Ingredients:

1 cup pumpkin puree

2 eggs

½ cup oats

2 cups whole wheat flour

3 tbsp peanut butter

Instructions:

Preheat oven to 350 degrees. In large mixing bowl, stir together pumpkin, eggs, and peanut butter. Mix in oats and flour. Stir well to form a sticky dough. Roll out dough on floured surface to ½ inch thickness. Cut into small shapes. Bake on parchment paper lined baking sheet for 30 minutes or until golden brown.

Sweet Potato Training Bites

Ingredients:

1 cup pureed sweet potato, canned or fresh cooked

1 ¾ cup whole wheat flour

1 egg

Instructions:

Preheat oven to 350 degrees. Mix all ingredients in mixing bowl. Place small balls of dough on parchment paper lined baking sheet. Press dough balls to flatten. Bake until golden brown.

Apple Carrot Training Bites

Ingredients:

1 egg

½ cup unsweetened apple sauce

1 cup carrots, grated

1 cup whole wheat flour

Instructions:

Preheat oven to 350 degrees. Mix all ingredients in mixing bowl. Place small balls of dough on parchment paper lined baking sheet. Press dough balls to flatten. Bake until golden brown.

Ginger Apple Training Bites

Ingredients:

1 cup brown rice or oat flour

½ cup apple, finely diced

2/3 cup greek yogurt

1 tsp fresh ginger, minced

1 tbsp coconut oil

Instructions:

Preheat oven to 350 degrees. Combine all ingredients, stir well. On a floured surface, roll dough to ¼ inch thick. Cut into small shapes. Bake on parchment paper lined baking sheet for 25 minutes.

Cinnamon Apple Training Treats

Ingredients:

1 cup quick cooking oatmeal

½ cup cinnamon apple sauce

1 egg

Instructions:

Preheat oven to 350 degrees. Mix all ingredients. Stir well. Drop small balls of dough onto parchment lined baking sheet. Bake for 20-25 minutes.

Pumpkin Training Bites

Ingredients:

1 cup whole grain flour, wheat flour, oat flour, ect

4 ounces pureed pumpkin

Instructions:

Preheat oven to 350 degrees. Combine ingredients in mixing bowl to form a stuff dough. If dough is too sticky, add flour. If dough is too dry, add water or pumpkin sparingly until workable. Lightly flour work area, roll dough to ¼ inch thick, and cut out small shapes with cookie cutters. On parchment paper lined baking sheet, bake cookies for 20-25 minutes. Allow to cool, serve fresh or store in freezer for prolonged storage.

Banana Training Bites

Ingredients:

1 cup whole grain flour, wheat flour, oat flour, ect

4 ounces mashed banana

Instructions:

Preheat oven to 350 degrees. Combine ingredients in mixing bowl to form a stuff dough. If dough is too sticky, add flour. If dough is too dry, add water or banana sparingly until workable. Lightly flour work area, roll dough to ¼ inch thick, and cut out small shapes with cookie cutters. On parchment paper lined baking sheet, bake cookies for 20-25 minutes. Allow to cool, serve fresh or store in freezer for prolonged storage.

Apple Training Bites

Ingredients:

1 cup whole grain flour, wheat flour, oat flour, ect

4 ounces unsweetened apple sauce

Instructions:

Preheat oven to 350 degrees. Combine ingredients in mixing bowl to form a stuff dough. If dough is too sticky, add flour. If dough is too dry, add water or applesauce sparingly until workable. Lightly flour work area, roll dough to ¼ inch thick, and cut out small shapes with cookie cutters. On parchment paper lined baking sheet, bake cookies for 20-25 minutes. Allow to cool, serve fresh or store in freezer for prolonged storage.

2 Ingredient Training Bites

Ingredients:

1 cup whole grain flour, wheat flour, oat flour, ect

4 ounces choice of pureed fruit or vegetable

Instructions:

Preheat oven to 350 degrees. Combine ingredients in mixing bowl to form a stuff dough. If dough is too sticky, add flour. If dough is too dry, add water or puree

sparingly until workable. Lightly flour work area, roll dough to ¼ inch thick, and cut out small shapes with cookie cutters. On parchment paper lined baking sheet, bake cookies for 20-25 minutes. Allow to cool, serve fresh or store in freezer for prolonged storage.

Pumpkin Peanut Butter Training Bites

Ingredients

1 cup canned pumpkin

½ cup peanut butter

1 ¾ cup whole wheat flour

Instructions:

Preheat oven to 350 degrees. Combine ingredients in mixing bowl to form a stuff dough. If dough is too sticky, add flour. If dough is too dry, add water or pumpkin sparingly until workable. Lightly flour work area, roll dough to ¼ inch thick, and cut out small shapes with cookie cutters. On parchment paper lined baking sheet, bake cookies for 10 minutes. Allow to cool, serve fresh or store in freezer for prolonged storage.

Mini Pig Trail Mix

1 cup raw whole almonds

1 cup raw pumpkin seeds

1 cup black oil sunflower seeds

1 cup mix nuts, unsalted (almonds, peanut, walnuts, brazil nuts, cashews, hazelnuts, macadamia nuts, pine nuts)

1 cup banana chips

Instructions:

Combine all ingredients. Can be used as a snack, training treats, or as a dish topping for any recipe. Store in airtight container and use as appropriate.

Mini Pig Seed Mix

Ingredients:

1 cup black oil sunflower seeds

1 cup raw pumpkin seeds

1 cup sesame seeds

1 cup chia seeds

1 cup quinoa

Instructions:

Combine all ingredients, dry. Can be used as a snack, training treats, or as a dish topping for any recipe. Store in airtight container and use as appropriate.

Air Popped Popcorn

Pop corn kernels in a hot air popcorn popper. Do not use oils, butter, or flavorings. The only ingredient should be corn. This can be stored in a bag or sealed container for 1 week or more. Great training treat!! We always travel with popcorn for a quick snack or distraction as needed. Simple, quick, and shelf stable. Popcorn Poppers are available at local stores or on Amazon.com for around $15.

Oatmeal

Plain oatmeal, old fashioned oats, or rolled oats can be given dry, scattered in the yard, scattered on the floor, or placed into a treat ball. Can also be warmed up with water and cooked for a meal. Add a dollop of yogurt and fruit for a special touch.

Cereal

Healthy cereals such as Cheerios, Shredded Wheat, and other whole grain cereals without added sugars make an excellent snack for training or on the go.

Dried Fruits and Vegetables

Can be dehydrated in oven or food dehydrator. Drying times will vary based on moisture content, thickness of slices, and temperature used. Foods may be peeled or leave skin on. Place slices of fruits/veggies on flat pan with parchment paper if placing in oven. Average drying time is 8-30 hours around 135 degrees with door propped open just a bit for 12-24 hours or until dried. If your oven goes above 200 then it may cook the food instead of dehydrating. Be sure to dry fruits and vegetables thoroughly. Foods must be sliced very thin, usually 1/8 inch to ¼ inch to dry through. Oven temperature should be low enough or the food may cook instead of dehydrating. Propping the oven door open a couple inches will help circulate the air and keep it from overheating. Once dried, store in air tight containers out of sunlight. If foods are not thoroughly dried, they will mold. Dehydrated foods can also be stored in the freezer to prolong freshness.

Perfect training treats for on the go. Healthy & mess free. No artificial chemicals or preservatives. Foods can be pre-treated before dehydrated if you choose.

Sweet Potato Chews

Slice sweet potatoes thinly. Arrange slices on a flat pan with parchment paper. Bake at 200-250 degrees for 3 hours.

Apple Chips

Core and slice apple thinly. Discard core. Place slices of apple on flat pan with parchment paper and follow "Dried Fruits and Vegetables" instructions.

Pumpkin Chips

Slice pumpkin thinly. Feed seeds & pumpkin guts to pigs or save for later Arrange slices on a flat pan with parchment paper and follow "Dried Fruits and Vegetables" instructions.

Banana Chips

Peel and slice banana thinly. Feed peels to pigs. Place slices of bananas on flat pan with parchment paper and follow "Dried Fruits and Vegetables" instructions.

Strawberry Chips

Cut tops off strawberries, feed tops to pigs. Slice strawberries thinly. Arrange slices on a flat pan with parchment paper and follow "Dried Fruits and Vegetables" instructions.

Beet Chips

Slice beets thinly. Feed beet tops to pigs or save for later. Arrange slices on a flat pan with parchment paper and follow "Dried Fruits and Vegetables" instructions.

Zucchini Chips

Slice zucchini thinly Arrange slices on a flat pan with parchment paper and follow "Dried Fruits and Vegetables" instructions.

Papaya

Cut open papaya. Save seeds for later or feed directly to pigs. Slice thin pieces of fruit, skin is fine too. Arrange slices on a flat pan with parchment paper and follow "Dried Fruits and Vegetables" instructions.

Mango

Cut mango into thin slices. Discard the pit. Arrange slices on a flat pan with parchment paper. Arrange slices on a flat pan with parchment paper and follow "Dried Fruits and Vegetables" instructions.

Pineapple

Place small chunks or slices of pineapple on flat pan with parchment paper and follow instructions above.

Acorn Squash

Slice acorn squash thinly. Feed seeds to pigs or save for later. Arrange slices on a flat pan with parchment paper and follow "Dried Fruits and Vegetables" instructions.

Butternut Squash

Slice butternut squash thinly. Feed seeds to
pigs or save for later. Arrange slices on a
flat pan with parchment paper and follow
"Dried Fruits and Vegetables" instructions.

Tomatoes

Slice tomatoes thinly. Arrange slices on a
flat pan with parchment paper and follow
"Dried Fruits and Vegetables" instructions.

CHAPTER 19

VITAMINS & SUPPLEMENTS

Coconut Oil Treats

Ingredients:

Coconut oil, unrefined & melted

Instructions:

Pour melted coconut oil into silicone molds or ice cube trays. Refrigerate or freeze until coconut oil solidifies. Store in fridge or freeze. Serve one treat per day.

Coconut Peppermint Breath Mints

Ingredients:

½ cup coconut oil, unrefined & melted

2-5 Drops of peppermint oil

Instructions:

In some measuring cup, stir together peppermint oil and coconut oil. Pour into silicone mold or ice cube tray. Refrigerate until solid. Store in fridge or freezer. Serve up to 1 treat daily.

Healthy Skin Treat

Ingredients:

Coconut oil, unrefined & melted

Fish Oil Capsules

Brewer's Yeast

Wheat Germ

Instructions:

Pour melted coconut oil into silicone molds or ice cube trays. Sprinkle a pinch of brewer's yeast and wheat germ over each treat. Drop one fish oil capsule into each treat. Refrigerate or freeze until coconut oil solidifies. Store in fridge or freeze. Serve one treat per day.

Coconut Cranberry Treat

Ingredients:

Coconut Oil, unrefined & melted

Cranberries, fresh or frozen

Instructions:

Pour melted coconut oil into silicone molds or ice cube trays. Drop 1 cranberry into each treat. Refrigerate until coconut oil solidifies. Store in fridge or freeze. Serve one treat daily.

Nutrient Dense Daily Treat

Ingredients:

Coconut oil, unrefined & melted

Wheat germ

Instructions:

Pour melted coconut oil into silicone molds or ice cube trays. Sprinkle wheat germ over each treat. Refrigerate until coconut oil solidifies. Store in fridge or freeze. Serve one treat daily.

Urinary Health Coconut Drops

Ingredients:

Coconut Oil, unrefined & melted

Cranberries, fresh or frozen

D-Mannose supplement powder

Instructions:

Pour melted coconut oil into silicone molds or ice cube trays. Sprinkle 1 tsp D-mannose powder over each treat. Drop 1 cranberry into each treat. Refrigerate until coconut oil solidifies. Store in fridge or freeze. Serve one treat twice daily.

Urinary Health Quencher

Ingredients:

¼ cup Apple Cider Vinegar, unrefined

¼ cup cranberry juice

½ cucumber, sliced

2 cups water

1 tsp D-Mannose supplement powder

Instructions:

Combine all ingredients. Serve chilled.

Super Foods Coconut Drops

Ingredients:

Coconut oil, unrefined & melted

Chia seeds

Flax seeds, ground

Brewer's yeast

Instructions:

Pour melted coconut oil into silicone molds or ice cube trays. Sprinkle chia seeds, flax seed, and brewer's yeast over each treat. Refrigerate until coconut oil solidifies. Store in fridge or freeze. Serve one treat twice daily.

Anti-inflammatory Coconut Drops

Ingredients:

Coconut oil, unrefined & melted

Yucca root powder

MSM supplement powder, pure

Tumeric root powder

Fish oil pills

Instructions:

Pour melted coconut oil into silicone molds or ice cube trays. Sprinkle yucca root, turmeric root, and MSM powders over each treat. Drop one fish oil pill in each treat. Refrigerate until coconut oil solidifies. Store in fridge or freezer. Serve one treat twice daily.

Anti-inflammatory Yogurt Bowl

Ingredients:

¼ cup yogurt, plain

1 tsp yucca root powder

1 tsp MSM supplement powder, pure

1 tsp turmeric root powder

1 tsp Fish oil pill

¼ cup oats

Instructions:

In serving dish or bowl, spread yogurt. Sprinkle yucca, MSM, and turmeric on yogurt. Top with oats and fish oil pill. Serve fresh.

Digestive Health Bowl

Ingredients:

¼ - ½ cup canned pumpkin

¼ cup apple cider vinegar, unrefined

1 tsp ginger root powder

1 tsp slippery elm

1 tsp yucca root powder

Instructions:

Mix all ingredients. Serve fresh.

Digestive Health Frozen Pop

Ingredients:

¼ - ½ cup canned pumpkin

ginger root powder

marshmallow root powder

yucca root powder

Rolled oats

Instructions:

Spoon canned pumpkin into silicone molds or ice cube trays. Sprinkle ginger, marshmallow, and yucca root powders over each treat. Top with rolled oats and press firmly into pumpkin mixture. Freeze until treats solidify. Store in freezer. Serve one treat daily.

Vitamin C Coconut Drops

Ingredients:

Coconut Oil, unrefined & melted

Cranberries, fresh or frozen

Blueberries, fresh or frozen

Instructions:

Pour melted coconut oil into silicone molds or ice cube trays. Drop 1 cranberry and 1 blueberry into each treat. Refrigerate until coconut oil solidifies. Store in fridge or freeze. Serve one treat each day.

Vitamin E & Selenium Booster

Ingredients:

½ cup canned Pumpkin

½ cup coconut oil, unrefined & melted

Chia seeds

Black oil sunflower seeds

Wheat germ

Almonds

Instructions:

Combine canned pumpkin and coconut oil. Press into silicone molds or ice cube trays. Sprinkle chia seeds, sunflower seeds, and wheat germ, then pressing one almond into each treat. Freeze until solid. Store in freezer. Serve one treat daily.

Daily Fiber Booster

Ingredients:

Canned pumpkin

Chia seeds

Flax seeds

Wheat bran

Rolled oats

Instructions:

Press canned pumpkin into silicone molds or ice cube trays. Sprinkle chia seeds, flax seeds, and wheat bran, then pressing rolled oats into each treat. Freeze until solid. Store in freezer. Serve one treat daily.

Hair & Hoof Health

Ingredients:

Coconut oil, unrefined and melted

1 biotin pill or gummy, 1,000 mcg

1 fish oil pill

1 vitamin c pill or gummy

Wheat germ

Instructions:

Pour melted coconut oil into silicone molds or ice cube trays. Sprinkle wheat germ over each treat. Drop biotin, fish oil, and vitamin c into each treat. Refrigerate until coconut oil solidifies. Store in fridge or freeze. Serve one treat each day.

Good Night Sleep Treat

Ingredients:

Canned pumpkin

Pumpkin seeds, raw

Valerian root powder

Rolled oats

Instructions:

Press pumpkin into silicone molds or ice cube trays. Sprinkle valerian root, rolled oats, and pumpkin seeds. Press firmly into pumpkin mixture. Freeze until solid. Store in fridge or freeze. Serve one treat each day.

Fall Superfoods Treat

Ingredients:

Canned pumpkin

Wheat Germ

Cranberry, fresh or frozen

Oats

Instructions:

Press pumpkin into silicone molds or ice cube trays. Sprinkle wheat germ, oats, and one cranberry into each treat. Press firmly into pumpkin mixture. Freeze until solid. Store in fridge or freeze. Serve one treat each day.

Tummy Soothing Treat

Ingredients:

Canned pumpkin

Grated ginger root

Peppermint leaves, chopped

Instructions:

Press pumpkin into silicone molds or ice cube trays. Sprinkle grated ginger root and peppermint leaves onto each treat. Press firmly into pumpkin mixture. Freeze until solid. Store in fridge or freeze. Serve one treat each day.

Appetite Kick Starter Treat

Ingredients:

½ cup canned pumpkin

½ cup coconut oil, melted and unrefined

Ginger, powder or freshy grated roots

Yucca root powder

Peppermint leaves, chopped

Instructions:

Stir together pumpkin and coconut oil. Press mixture into silicone molds or ice cube trays. Sprinkle grated ginger root and peppermint leaves onto each treat. Press firmly into pumpkin mixture. Freeze until solid. Store in fridge or freeze. Serve one treat each day.

CHAPTER 20

NATURAL BUG REPELLENTS

Natural Flea and Tick Repellant for Pigs, Pets, and Kids

Ingredients:

8 oz apple cider vinegar

4 oz warm water

1/2 tsp salt

1/2 tsp baking soda

Instructions:

First mix dry ingredients. Then slowly add to wet as the vinegar and baking soda will react slightly. Store in spray bottle. Safe for mini pigs, other pets, and children. Avoid eye, nose, and mouth areas.

Apple Cider Vinegar

ACV is said to add acidity to your mini pig's blood making it less appetizing to fleas and ticks. Add 2 tablespoons of the apple cider vinegar to your mini pig's food or water as a flea and tick preventative.

Basic Vinegar Spritz

Ingredients:

1 cup white vinegar

1 cup water

Instructions:

Mix ingredients well, place in spray bottle. Spritz directly onto mini pig avoiding the eyes.

Flea and Tick Spritz

Ingredients:

1 cup white vinegar

1 cup water

2 tablespoons almond oil

1 tablespoon lemon juice

Instructions:

Mix ingredients well, place in spray bottle. Spritz directly onto mini pig avoiding the eyes.

Flea/Tick "Collar"

Since collars are not safe for mini pigs, this recipe may be adjusted to be used on your pet's harness, velcro a bandana around their neck, or have the pig wear a tshirt. This recipe will only be useful while your mini pig is wearing the harness or clothing, which is great for hiking or camping.

Mix 2 tablespoons of Almond Oil with Rose Geranium Oil, Palo Santo, or your choice of Essential Oils (EO). Spray or dab onto chosen item. Alternately, Essential Oils may be applied directly to chosen item (harness, bandana, or clothing).

Citrus Repellent

Cut one lemon, lime, orange, or grapefruit into quarters and put into a glass jar. Cover with boiling water. Let steep overnight. Pour the liquid into a spray bottle.This can be sprayed directly on the mini pig, on their clothing, bedding, and yard areas. Avoid the face and eyes.

Alternate Version:

Boil 2 cups of water. Add 2 sliced citrus fruits: lemons, limes, oranges, or grapefruit Boil for about a minute, then simmer for one hour. Remove the fruit Pour into a spray bottle Safe for skin, clothing, bedding, and yard.

Diatomaceous Earth

Food Grade Diatomaceous Earth (DE) can be used to prevent fleas and ticks. Sprinkle DE at the rate of 1 pound per 1,000 sq feet of yard. This can be sprinkled in areas that pigs will graze (it is safe to eat), on their bedding, in their enclosure, in their straw or hay, inside the home, or even directly on the mini pig's skin, although it is drying. DE is ineffective once wet. It will need to be reapplied after rain or wind in order to be effective.

Essential Oil Tick Repellent – Water Based

Ingredients:

2 ounces Apple Cider Vinegar or Witch Hazel

2 ounces water

30-40 drops of Geranium Oil OR your choice of EO

1/4 teaspoon castile soap (optional) to distribute oil in water

Instructions:

Mix EOs with Apple Cider Vinegar or Witch Hazel, then add water. Mix well. Put into spray bottle. Store in fridge and shake well before use. Spritz on skin or clothing. Avoid eye contact.

Essential Oil Tick Repellent – Oil Based

Ingredients:

4 ounces oil (almond oil, olive oil, jajoba oil)

30-40 drops Geranium Oil OR your choice of EO

Instructions:

Mix oil with EOs in spray bottle. Store in fridge. Shake well before use. Spritz onto skin or clothing. Avoid eye contact.

Essential Oil Tick Repellent – Lotion

Ingredients:

2 ounces of unscented lotion

20 to 40 drops of Geranium Oil OR your choice of EO.

Instructions:

Combine ingredients, apply as desired.

Parasite Dust

Ingredients:

1 part powdered Rosemary

1 part powdered Rue

1 part powdered Wormwood

Instructions:

Mix ingredients in equal parts. Dust the mini pig with Parasite Dust before tick infested ventures. Store in a jar with a shaker lid in a cool, dry, dark place.

Rose Geranium Oil

Ingredients:

1-3 drops of Rose Geranium oil

Instructions:

Place between the shoulder blades of your mini pig.

Fragranced Apple Cider Vinegar

Ingredients:

1 cup water

1/2 cup Apple Cider Vinegar (ACV)

10 drops Geranium Oil or your choice of Eos

Instructions:

Put into spray bottle and spritz your mini pig directly, their clothing, their yard, or enclosure.

Flea Repellant Rosemary Rinse

Ingredients:

1 cup fresh rosemary leaves

1 quart water

Instructions:

Boil rosemary leaves in water. Allow to boil for 5 minutes then turn off heat and cover pot until cooled. Store in air tight bottle. Use as a flea fighting conditioning rinse.

Flea Fighting Shampoo

Ingredients:

1 quart water

1 cup white vinegar or apple cider vinegar

1 cup Dawn dish soap

Instructions:

Mix ingredients together. Use to wash mini pig, then rinse well.

Bug Bite Itch No More Sticks

Ingredients:

1 tbsp beeswax

3 tbsp calendula infused oil

6 drops peppermint essential oil

3 drops lavender essential oil

1 drop tea tree essential oil

6 lip balm tubes

Instructions:

Using a double broiler, warm beeswax and oil. Heat until melted. Remove from heat, add essential oils. Pour mixture into lip balm tubes. Allow to cool. Use on bug bites, itches, and minor scrapes.

Bug Repellent Lotion Bars

Ingredients:

1 Tbls. Beeswax

4 Tbls. Shea butter

2 Tbls. Coconut oil

10 drops citronella oil

5 drops peppermint essential oil

5 drops lemon essential oil

20 drops lemongrass essential oil

Soap mold or muffin tin

Instructions:

Melt together beeswax, shea butter, and coconut oil in a double broiler or microwave safe bow.

Add the essential oils and mix well.

Pour mixture into soap molds or muffin tin and allow to cool. You can speed up the cooling process by placing in the refrigerator. When bars are solid, remove from mold and store in an airtight container.

Bug Repellant Balm

Ingredients:

¼ cup coconut oil

1/8 cup shea butter

4 teas. Beeswax granules

12 drops citronella essential oil

8 drops rosemary essential oil

8 drops cedarwood essential oil

8 drops lemongrass essential oil

8 drops eucalyptus or tea tree essential oil

Jars for storage

Instructions:

Prepare a double boiler by bringing water to a boil and then lowering heat to med-low. Add coconut oil and shea butter and melt while stirring. Add beeswax and mix until blended and well melted.

Remove from heat and let cool for 3-5 minutes and then whisk in the essential oils until thoroughly combined.

Poor the liquid into storage jars and let cool at room temperature, before adding lids.

Once completely cooled, place the lids on for storage.

CHAPTER 21

SKIN CARE RECIPES

Mini Pig Skin & Hair Premium Conditioner

Ingredients:

2 tbsp coconut oil

1 tbsp argon oil

1 tbsp honey

4 drops lavender essential oil

Instructions:

Mix ingredients together. Massage onto mini pig, let soak for 5 minutes or more, then rinse.

Natural Coconut Oil Body Butter for Skin and Hair

Ingredients:

1 cup Coconut oil

Optional:

A few drops of your favorite Essential Oils

Instructions:

Place solid (not melted) coconut oil into food mixer. Mix on high speed with wire whisk attachment until it reaches a whipped, airy consistency. Spoon whipped coconut oil into jar(s). Store at room temperature. If house temperature is high enough to melt the oil, store in refrigerator to maintain the whipped texture. This recipe yields a fluffy whipped coconut oil that can be easily massaged onto your pig after bath time!

Coconut Oil Peppermint Sugar Scrub to Exfoliate Dry Skin

Ingredients:

1/2 cup sugar

1/2 cup coconut oil

10-20 drop of peppermint oil (optional)

Instructions:

Combine all ingredients mixing well. Store in airtight jar or container for up to two months.

Oatmeal Coconut Conditioner

Ingredients:

3 tbsp coconut oil

1/3 cup oatmeal (grind in blender or food processor)

1 tbsp honey

2 drops Lavender essential oil

Instructions:

Mix ingredients together. Massage onto mini pig, let soak for 5 minutes or more, then rinse.

Gentle Mini Pig Shampoo

Ingredients:

1/2 cup liquid Castile soap

1/4 cup white vinegar or apple cider vinegar

1 tbsp olive oil

2 tbsp water

Instructions:

Combine all ingredients in lidded bottle. Gently shake the bottle to mix ingredients prior to shampooing mini pig. Rinse mini pig well after shampoo.

Rosemary Coconut Oil Conditioning Shampoo

Ingredients:

3 cups water

3 rosemary stems

1 tbsp coconut oil, melted

5 tbsp Dr. Bronner's Baby-mild liquid soap

4 drops Lavender essential oil

Instructions:

Bring water to a boil. Drop rosemary stems into water. Cover pot and turn off heat. Allow to steep until cooled. Discard rosemary stems. Pour rosemary infused water into bottle. Pour in all other ingredients. Gently shake the bottle to mix ingredients prior to shampooing the mini pig. Rinse mini pig well after shampoo.

Natural Oatmeal Shampoo

Ingredients:

1 cup plain oatmeal

1/2 cup baking soda

1 quart warm water

Instructions:

In food processor, blender, or coffee grinder, gnd oatmeal until powdered. In container, mix together powdered oatmeal and baking soda. Add warm water and stir until mixed well. Use as shampoo, massaging into skin and hair. Rinse well.

Coconut Milk Shampoo

Ingredients:

¼ cup coconut milk

1/3 cup castile soap

½ teaspoon vitamin E oil

10-20 drops of your favorite essential oils (optional)

Instructions:

Mix the ingredients in an old, well cleaned shampoo bottle.

Shake before each use. Massage on for one minute before rinsing.

Mini Pig Dry Skin Polish

Ingredients:

1/2 ground rice (grind in blender or food processor)

1/2 cup coconut milk

1/4 cup brown sugar

1 1/2 tbsp ground ginger

Instructions:

Mix ingredients to form a healing paste. Massage paste in circular motion on dry areas of skin to exfoliate and soothe. Store in air tight jar.

Easy Mini Pig Whipped Beauty Crème

Ingredients:

1/3 cup coconut oil

1/3 cup shea butter

10 drops lavender or your favorite essential oil. (orange, lemon, grapefruit are wonderful!)

Small mason jars or airtight containers

Instructions:

Soften shea butter in the microwave for 30 seconds.

Mix in room temperature coconut oil with a hand mixer for 15 minutes or until the oils are fluffy.

Add essential oils and mix well. Transfer to mason jars or storage containers.

Whipped Peppermint Body Butter

Ingredients:

½ cup coconut oil

½ cup cocoa butter

½ cup shea butter

½ cup sweet almond oil

1 tsp vitamin E oil

2-4 drops of peppermint essential oils (or replace with your favorite essential oil)

Instructions:

Place coconut oil, cocoa butter, and shea butter in a pot on low heat or in a microwave safe bowl. Heat and stir until melted.

Add and mix in the sweet almond oil, vitamin E, and peppermint oil.

Chill in the refrigerator for an hour or until the mixture is firm, but not solid.

Once chilled mix with hand mixer on high until whipped.

Scoop into a mason jar or small containers for storing.

Mini Pig Lotion Bar

Ingredients:

1 cup Shea Butter

1 cup Cocoa butter

1 cup Organic Beeswax pellets

1 teas. Vitamin E oil

30 drops of your preferred essential oils (orange, lavender, lemon, lime, orange, grapefruit)

Soap Mold, plastic food storage container lined with wax paper, silicone muffin or loaf pan

Instructions:

Melt the first three ingredients in a glass mixing bowl in the microwave or in a double broiler or candle making pitcher, stirring well.

Once melted and combined well, add the vitamin E and essential oils.

Carefully pour your lotion mixture into your mold. Allow to cool or cool in the refrigerator or freezer.

Once cooled, remove bars from the molds. Cut bars if need and they are ready for use.

Silky Smooth Mini Pig Lotion

Ingredients:

¾ cup sweet almond oil

1 tsp Vitamin E oil

3 tablespoons refined mango butter

2 tablespoons cocoa butter

1 tablespoon beeswax pellets

1 cup distilled water

20-40 drops lavender or orange essential oils

Pump bottle container for dispensing this fine lotion. Jar for storing excess.

Instructions:

Combine sweet almond oil, mango butter, cocoa butter, and beeswax in a clean, heat safe bowl. Microwave in 30 second intervals stirring well, or use a double boiler to melt and combine.

Once combined, let the mixture cool to room temperature, but no solid. Add vitamin E and the essential oil into the cooled mixture. Use a mixer or blender to pulse mix a few times.

Slowly add the distilled water while mixing at medium for 30 seconds. Pour the lotion into a jar for storage. Let it rest for 24 hours before using in your pump bottle dispenser.

Pig's Love Pumpkin Moisturizing Lotion

Ingredients:

¼ cup cocoa butter

2 tablespoons almond oil

2 tablespoons coconut oil

1 teaspoon beeswax

1/8-1/4 teaspoon paprika for color

10 drops cinnamon essential oil

7 drops ginger essential oil

5 drops nutmeg essential oil

2 drops allspice essential oil

2 drops clove essential oil

Instructions:

Mix cocoa butter, coconut oil, almond oil and beeswax in a bowl and melt in microwave in 30 second intervals while stirring or use a double boiler to melt and combined.

Once melted and combined thoroughly add paprika and let seep for 10 minutes for color.

If the paprika does not dissolve completely drain off by pouring the melted oils into a clean bowl leaving the undissolved paprika behind.

Place the bowl in the refrigerator to cool.

When the lotion is almost solid, but not completely solid, remove from the refrigerator. Add essential oils and whip with a hand mixer until fluffy.

Transfer to jars for storage. Your lotion is ready for use immediately.

Honey Oatmeal Goatmilk Soap

Ingredients:

1 /2 lb Suspension Soap Base Goats Milk (Available at amazon.com)

2 tbsp honey

2 1/2 tbsp oats

Instructions:

Use blender or coffee grinder to grind 2 tbsps oats into a powder. Set aside other 1/2 tbsp oats. Cut 1/2 lb soap base into cubes. Microwave in a glass measuring cup stirring at 30-second increments, until melted. Do not overheat. Stir thoroughly to melt smaller pieces of soap. Gently stir in honey and powdered oats.

Sprinkle remaining oats into silicone molds. Pour soap into silicone molds evenly. Allow to cool and harden. Use the soap for people and pigs!

Lavender and Goat's Milk Soap

Ingredients:

2 lbs. of Goat's Milk Soap Base Melt & Pour

Lavendar Essential Oil

Soap Coloring(optional)

Dried Lavender Flowers

Silicone Mold

Instructions:

Cut the Goat's Milk base into cubes. Melt in the microwave in 30 second increments, stirring well.

Once thoroughly melted, add 10 drops of soap coloring (optional). Then add 15-20 drops of Lavender Essential Oil and dried lavender flowers.

Pour into the soap mold and let sit for 45 minutes to cool. Once completely cooled, remove from molds and your soap is ready to use.

Rosemary Citrus Goats Milk Soap

Ingredients:

½ pd. Goats Milk Soap Base

Citrus or Orange Essential Oils

Fresh Rosemary chopped

Grated rind from 2 small oranges

Instructions:

Cut the goats milk soap base into cubes and melt in the microwave in 30 second increments, stirring well.

Once melted, stir in the chopped rosemary. Add as much or as little as you would like to get the desired look.

Add the grated orange rind and 10-15 drops of citrus essential oil. Stir well.

Pour soap into the molds and allow to cool. Once completely cooled, carefully remove from molds and your soap is ready to use.

Exfoliating Coffee and Milk Soap

Ingredients:

2 lbs of Goats Milk soap base melt & pour

Coffee grounds

Coffee Essential Oil

Soap mold

Instructions:

Cut the soap base into cubes and melt in the microwave in 30 second increments, stirring well.

Once thoroughly melted, add coffee grounds, as much or as little as needed to get the desired effect.

Add 15 drops of coffee essential oil and stir well.

Pour the soap mixture into the molds and allow to cool.

Once completely cooled, carefully remove soap from the molds and your soap is ready to use.

Whipped Coconut Oil Body Butter

Ingredients:

1 coconut oil (solid, cannot be melted)

Essential oils (optional)

Use mixer to whip solid coconut oil until the texture resembles whipped butter or whipped cream. Add in drops of essential oils if desired. Use to exfoliate dry flaky skin leaving it smooth and polished.

Simple Coconut Oil Sugar Scrub

Ingredients:

1 cup white sugar

1/4 cup coconut oil

Instructions:

Fold ingredients together. Store in airtight container. Use to exfoliate dry flaky skin leaving it smooth and polished.

Peppermint Hoof Scrub

Ingredients:

3/4 cup raw sugar

1/4 cup coconut oil

20 drops peppermint essential oil

Instructions:

Fold ingredients together. Place into airtight container, refrigerate for 30 minutes. Perfect to exfoliate and polish hooves and legs. This uses a much coarser sugar for more exfoliating power than the Face & Body Scrubs, avoid face or tender areas.

Citrus Face & Body Scrub

Ingredients:

1 cup white sugar

1/4 cup coconut oil

20 drops sweet orange essential oil

10 drops lemon essential oil

Instructions:

Fold ingredients together. Store in airtight container. Use to exfoliate dry flaky skin leaving it smooth and polished.

"Sleeping Beauty" Face & Body Scrub

Ingredients:

1 cup white sugar

1/4 cup coconut oil

15 drops lavender essential oil

5 drops patchouli oil

7 drops sweet orange essential oil

Instructions:

Fold ingredients together. Store in airtight container. Use to exfoliate dry flaky skin leaving it smooth and polished.

Vanilla Sugar Scrub

Ingredients:

1/2 cup brown sugar

1/2 cup white sugar

1/8 cup coconut oil

1/8 cup avocado oil or almond oil

1 tbsp honey

1 tsp vanilla extract

Instructions:

Fold ingredients together. Store in airtight container. Use to exfoliate dry flaky skin leaving it smooth and polished.

Lemon Sugar Scrub

Ingredients:

1 cup white sugar

1/4 cup coconut oil

10-20 drops lemon essential oil

Instructions:

Fold ingredients together. Store in airtight container. Use to exfoliate dry flaky skin leaving it smooth and polished.

Spay Day Pig Body Scrub

Ingredients:

1 cup white sugar

1/4 cup oil (mix together coconut oil, avocado oil, almond oil, and/or olive oil)

5-10 drops lavender essential oil

5-10 drops eucalyptus essential oil

5-10 drops peppermint

Instructions:

Fold ingredients together. Store in airtight container. Use to exfoliate dry flaky skin leaving it smooth and polished.

Cherry Almond Sugar Scrub

Ingredients:

1 cup white sugar

1/4 cup almond oil

1 tsp cherry extract

Instructions:

Fold ingredients together. Store in airtight container. Use to exfoliate dry flaky skin leaving it smooth and polished.

Cucumber Mint Sugar Scrub

Ingredients:

1 cup white sugar

1/4 cup olive oil

5 drops peppermint essential oil

5 drops cucumber essential oil

Instructions:

Fold ingredients together. Store in airtight container. Use to exfoliate dry flaky skin leaving it smooth and polished.

Honey & Brown Sugar Scrub

Ingredients:

1 cup brown sugar

1/4 cup olive oil

1 tsp vanilla extract

1 tsp honey

Instructions:

Fold ingredients together. Store in airtight container. Use to exfoliate dry flaky skin leaving it smooth and polished.

GIFT TAGS

Many of the recipes make excellent gifts for mini pig gift exchanges and for human friends and family. Enjoy these easy to use gift tags with ingredient lists.

Enjoy this AMPA Mini Pig Trail Mix homemade with love by:

The recipe can be found in **The AMPA's Ultimate Cookbook at www.americanminipigstore.com**

Ingredients: raw whole almonds, raw pumpkin seeds, black oil sunflower seeds, unsalted mix nuts, banana chips

Enjoy this AMPA Mini Pig Trail Mix homemade with love by:

The recipe can be found in **The AMPA's Ultimate Cookbook at www.americanminipigstore.com**

Ingredients: raw whole almonds, raw pumpkin seeds, black oil sunflower seeds, unsalted mix nuts, banana chips

Enjoy this AMPA Mini Pig Trail Mix homemade with love by:

The recipe can be found in **The AMPA's Ultimate Cookbook at www.americanminipigstore.com**

Ingredients: raw whole almonds, raw pumpkin seeds, black oil sunflower seeds, unsalted mix nuts, banana chips

Enjoy this AMPA Mini Pig Trail Mix homemade with love by:

The recipe can be found in **The AMPA's Ultimate Cookbook at www.americanminipigstore.com**

Ingredients: raw whole almonds, raw pumpkin seeds, black oil sunflower seeds, unsalted mix nuts, banana chips

Enjoy this AMPA Ultimate Training Mix is homemade with love by:

The recipe can be found in The AMPA's Ultimate Cookbook at www.americanminipigstore.com

Ingredients: unsalted mixed nuts, unsalted almonds (optional), black oil sunflower seeds, unsalted pumpkin seeds, dried coconut chunks, dried strawberry slices

Enjoy this AMPA Ultimate Training Mix is homemade with love by:

The recipe can be found in The AMPA's Ultimate Cookbook at www.americanminipigstore.com

Ingredients: unsalted mixed nuts, unsalted almonds (optional), black oil sunflower seeds, unsalted pumpkin seeds, dried coconut chunks, dried strawberry slices

Enjoy this AMPA Ultimate Training Mix is homemade with love by:

The recipe can be found in The AMPA's Ultimate Cookbook at www.americanminipigstore.com

Ingredients: unsalted mixed nuts, unsalted almonds (optional), black oil sunflower seeds, unsalted pumpkin seeds, dried coconut chunks, dried strawberry slices

Enjoy this AMPA Ultimate Training Mix is homemade with love by:

The recipe can be found in The AMPA's Ultimate Cookbook at www.americanminipigstore.com

Ingredients: unsalted mixed nuts, unsalted almonds (optional), black oil sunflower seeds, unsalted pumpkin seeds, dried coconut chunks, dried strawberry slices

Enjoy this AMPA Mini Pig Whipped Beauty Crème *is homemade with love by:*

The recipe can be found in The AMPA's Ultimate Cookbook at www.americanminipigstore.com

Ingredients: coconut oil, shea butter, essential oils

Enjoy this AMPA Mini Pig Whipped Beauty Crème *is homemade with love by:*

The recipe can be found in The AMPA's Ultimate Cookbook at www.americanminipigstore.com

Ingredients: coconut oil, shea butter, essential oils

Enjoy this AMPA Mini Pig Whipped Beauty Crème *is homemade with love by:*

The recipe can be found in The AMPA's Ultimate Cookbook at www.americanminipigstore.com

Ingredients: coconut oil, shea butter, essential oils

Enjoy this AMPA Mini Pig Whipped Beauty Crème *is homemade with love by:*

The recipe can be found in The AMPA's Ultimate Cookbook at www.americanminipigstore.com

Ingredients: coconut oil, shea butter, essential oils

Enjoy this AMPA Mini Pig Vanilla Sugar Scrub is homemade with love by:

The recipe can be found in The AMPA's Ultimate Cookbook at www.americanminipigstore.com

Ingredients: brown sugar, white sugar, coconut oil, avocado oil or almond oil, honey, vanilla extract

Enjoy this AMPA Mini Pig Vanilla Sugar Scrub is homemade with love by:

The recipe can be found in The AMPA's Ultimate Cookbook at www.americanminipigstore.com

Ingredients: brown sugar, white sugar, coconut oil, avocado oil or almond oil, honey, vanilla extract

Enjoy this AMPA Mini Pig Vanilla Sugar Scrub is homemade with love by:

The recipe can be found in The AMPA's Ultimate Cookbook at www.americanminipigstore.com

Ingredients: brown sugar, white sugar, coconut oil, avocado oil or almond oil, honey, vanilla extract

Enjoy this AMPA Mini Pig Vanilla Sugar Scrub is homemade with love by:

The recipe can be found in The AMPA's Ultimate Cookbook at www.americanminipigstore.com

Ingredients: brown sugar, white sugar, coconut oil, avocado oil or almond oil, honey, vanilla extract

Enjoy this AMPA Mini Pig Honey & Brown Sugar Scrub is homemade with love by:

The recipe can be found in The AMPA's Ultimate Cookbook at www.americanminipigstore.com

Ingredients: brown sugar, olive oil, vanilla extract, honey

Enjoy this AMPA Mini Pig Honey & Brown Sugar Scrub is homemade with love by:

The recipe can be found in The AMPA's Ultimate Cookbook at www.americanminipigstore.com

Ingredients: brown sugar, olive oil, vanilla extract, honey

Enjoy this AMPA Mini Pig Honey & Brown Sugar Scrub is homemade with love by:

The recipe can be found in The AMPA's Ultimate Cookbook at www.americanminipigstore.com

Ingredients: brown sugar, olive oil, vanilla extract, honey

Enjoy this AMPA Mini Pig Honey & Brown Sugar Scrub is homemade with love by:

The recipe can be found in The AMPA's Ultimate Cookbook at www.americanminipigstore.com

Ingredients: brown sugar, olive oil, vanilla extract, honey

Enjoy this AMPA Whipped Peppermint Body Butter is homemade with love by:

The recipe can be found in The AMPA's Ultimate Cookbook at www.americanminipigstore.com

Ingredients: coconut oil, cocoa butter, shea butter, sweet almond oil, vitamin E oil, peppermint essential oils

Enjoy this AMPA Whipped Peppermint Body Butter is homemade with love by:

The recipe can be found in The AMPA's Ultimate Cookbook at www.americanminipigstore.com

Ingredients: coconut oil, cocoa butter, shea butter, sweet almond oil, vitamin E oil, peppermint essential oils

Enjoy this AMPA Whipped Peppermint Body Butter is homemade with love by:

The recipe can be found in The AMPA's Ultimate Cookbook at www.americanminipigstore.com

Ingredients: coconut oil, cocoa butter, shea butter, sweet almond oil, vitamin E oil, peppermint essential oils

Enjoy this AMPA Whipped Peppermint Body Butter is homemade with love by:

The recipe can be found in The AMPA's Ultimate Cookbook at www.americanminipigstore.com

Ingredients: coconut oil, cocoa butter, shea butter, sweet almond oil, vitamin E oil, peppermint essential oils

Enjoy this AMPA Mini Pig gift, homemade with love by:

The recipe can be found in The AMPA's Ultimate Cookbook at www.americanminipigstore.com

Ingredients:

Enjoy this AMPA Mini Pig gift, homemade with love by:

The recipe can be found in The AMPA's Ultimate Cookbook at www.americanminipigstore.com

Ingredients:

Enjoy this AMPA Mini Pig gift, homemade with love by:

The recipe can be found in The AMPA's Ultimate Cookbook at www.americanminipigstore.com

Ingredients:

Enjoy this AMPA Mini Pig gift, homemade with love by:

The recipe can be found in The AMPA's Ultimate Cookbook at www.americanminipigstore.com

Ingredients:

Enjoy this AMPA Mini Pig gift, homemade with love by:

The recipe can be found in The AMPA's Ultimate Cookbook at www.americanminipigstore.com

Ingredients:

Enjoy this AMPA Mini Pig gift, homemade with love by:

The recipe can be found in The AMPA's Ultimate Cookbook at www.americanminipigstore.com

Ingredients:

Enjoy this AMPA Mini Pig gift, homemade with love by:

The recipe can be found in The AMPA's Ultimate Cookbook at www.americanminipigstore.com

Ingredients:

Enjoy this AMPA Mini Pig gift, homemade with love by:

The recipe can be found in The AMPA's Ultimate Cookbook at www.americanminipigstore.com

Ingredients: